Anaesthesia a

T.C.K. BROWN
MB, ChB, MD, FFARACS
Director of Anaesthesia
Royal Children's Hospital,
Melbourne

With a chapter on Electrical Hazards by
GLEN JOHNSTON
ARMIT

Foreword by
CLIFFORD C. BUCHANAN
SRN, DipNEd, DipNAdmin, FCNA
Director of Nursing
Repatriation General Hospital
Concord, NSW

BLACKWELL SCIENTIFIC PUBLICATIONS

MELBOURNE OXFORD LONDON
EDINBURGH BOSTON

© 1983 by
Blackwell Scientific Publications
Editorial offices:
99 Barry Street, Carlton
  Victoria 3053 Australia
Osney Mead, Oxford OX2 OEL
8 John Street, London WC1N 2ES
9 Forrest Road, Edinburgh EH1 2QH
52 Beacon Street, Boston
  Massachusetts 02108, USA

First published 1983

Typeset by ABB-Typesetting Pty Ltd

Printed in Hong Kong

DISTRIBUTORS

USA
  Blackwell Mosby Book Distributors
  11830 Westline Industrial Drive
  St Louis, Missouri 63141

Canada
  Blackwell Mosby Book Distributors
  120 Melford Drive, Scarborough
  Ontario M1B 2X4

Australia
  Blackwell Scientific Book Distributors
  214 Berkeley Street, Carlton
  Victoria 3053

Cataloguing in Publication Data
Brown, T.C.K.
  Anaesthesia and patient care
  Bibliography
  Includes index
  ISBN 0 86793 048 9
  1. Anesthesiology
  2. Patient monitoring
  I Johnston, Glen
  II. Title
617'.96

CONTENTS

FOREWORD

This book has been needed for a long time. It gives nurses a better under-standing of their role in relation to anaesthesia and also provides useful information for anaesthetic assistants and medical students having their initial exposure to anaesthesia. The subject of the care of the patient undergoing anaesthesia has rarely been accorded the detailed attention it deserves and requires; even more rarely has the subject been presented in the simple style that Kester Brown displays in the pages ahead.

Beyond the theory that we associate with the study of anaesthesia — physiology, drugs, equipment and safety, for example — we need to know more about the patient committed for surgery, the responsibility of the nurse and the roles of others involved in the care of the patient.

It is precisely because aspects of this nature are clearly addressed and explained that this is an important book and it is these dimensions of the book which, taken together, make it an extraordinary contribution to nursing students and nurse educators alike, and a valuable introduction for medical students and anaesthetic technicians to whom it is also addressed.

Sydney, 1982   Clifford C. Buchanan

PREFACE

This book has been written to provide a concise, practical introduction to anaesthesia and to outline the care of surgical patients, particularly in relation to anaesthesia and postanaesthetic recovery. It also provides information about anaesthetic equipment and how it is cleaned and sterilized. Basic principles of physiology, pharmacology, resuscitation and electrical safety are presented so that their application in the care of the patient having an anaesthetic can be appreciated. The specialized care of patients undergoing open heart surgery is beyond the scope of this book although most of the general principles outlined will apply to these patients.

It is hoped that this introduction to anaesthesia and the emphasis placed on the care of the patient undergoing anaesthesia will be easy to understand and will be of practical value to medical students, nurses and anaesthetic technicians.

Melbourne, 1982   Kester Brown

ACKNOWLEDGEMENTS

Many people have played a part in producing this book. My sister, who is a nurse, encouraged me during the first difficult stages of writing the first draft and Malcolm Dodd and Martin Schabet, as medical students, encouraged me to expand the text for medical students. Many nurses, medical students and anaesthetists have read and made useful comments on the text as it has developed. In particular, I would like to thank Pam Atkinson, who also contributed to the appendix on handling infected patients, Dr Geoff Tauro, Director of the Royal Children's Hospital Haematology Laboratory and Blood Bank, who gave me valuable assistance in preparing the section on blood transfusion, Heather Telfer, Noel Cass, Rod Westhorpe, Barbara Main, Mary Dwyer, Alan Duncan, John Paull and Ted Sumner for their ideas and constructive criticism.

Glen Johnston, recently retired head of the Hospital Electronics Department, contributed the chapter on Electrical Hazards. His lucid style which has helped so many nurses, doctors and technical staff in the past to understand electrical equipment and its applications will continue to do so through his chapter on the subject.

'A picture is worth a thousand words' — our Department of Medical Illustration is to be thanked for the fine set of illustrations they have prepared for the book as is Robyn Jones who drew the illustration on the cover. Figure 6.17 was produced at The Royal Women's Hospital specially for this book.

I am also grateful to my wife and family for their support during the time I spent writing the manuscript.

Finally but most importantly, I owe much gratitude to my secretary, Pamela Corden, for typing the manuscript and all the help she has given me during the preparation of this book.

CHAPTER 1

The patient

Surgery is a major event in the lives of most people. They may remember some events related to the operative period for the rest of their lives unless they are very young or so ill that they are unaware of the situation.

It is important to realize that most people are worried preoperatively. This may be because they fear that the operative findings may spell doom (e.g. cancer). They may fear disfigurement, pain, being sick post-operatively or even that they will let out some secret as they go under the anaesthetic (this is a very rare happening but is a real concern to some people). A bad experience with a previous anaesthetic is an aggravating factor. Patients should be encouraged to express these fears. Sometimes they find it difficult to discuss them with the surgeon either because they feel that he is too busy, lacking in sympathy or that they would be embarrassed. Sometimes the anaesthetist helps to allay these fears by asking questions and giving the person the chance to say what he or she is feeling, but there are some anaesthetists who find it difficult to communicate easily with their patients or whose visit is too brief to allow the patient much opportunity for discussion.

The nurse can have a very important supportive role to play because he or she will usually spend more time with the patient. A nurse who provides a listening ear, is understanding and shows compassion can provide reassurance to any patient about to undergo surgery and thereby reduce his anxiety. It must be remembered that even those patients who put on an apparently brave front may be apprehensive. Sweaty skin or collapsed peripheral veins due to high levels of circulating catechol-amines (adrenaline and noradrenaline) may be found in frightened people as well as those who have suffered loss of blood.

Children pose particular problems. Neonates are unaware of what is going to happen. As infants grow older and their maternal attachment grows stronger separation becomes more traumatic to the child and often to the mother who sometimes conveys her anxiety to the infant or 'small child, making it more difficult for her offspring. Children up to 3 or 4 years old suffer most from this separation. Older children tend to cope better, especially if procedures are explained to them beforehand in a way that they understand. A group which often hides its apprehension until the time of induction is boys of about 10 years.

Most parents do not like to see their children unhappy and crying. Racial and cultural differences may lead one parent to leave the child in hospital, not having told him or her about the operation and not return until the child is ready to go home, while another may wish to be with the child every minute of the hospitalization except during the actual surgery. The reasons for their behaviour may be similar but their actions are very different. Most parents fall between these extremes but both types of parent may be encountered.

Racial factors influence the way people react when they are going to have an operation. These must be recognized and accepted by the staff. Some races express their emotions verbally and physically much more than others who may show no apparent emotion, and yet both may have similar feelings. The difference often lies in the way people are brought up to react to situations and because a patient reacts differently to the way one feels he or she should behave, it is not reasonable to be critical or intolerant of the patient for doing so.

An awareness of the many factors influencing a patient's behaviour can help the staff to realize that each patient has to be dealt with as an individual. All require some caring attention and reassurance before an operation. Talking to the patient, especially if addressed by name, conveys a feeling that the staff are interested in him or her. Too much small talk with other staff while ignoring the presence of the patient will very quickly make the patient feel of secondary importance at a time when he or she needs the greatest support. Staff should be careful what they say within earshot of patients because inappropriate comments may be misconstrued and cause alarm.

CHAPTER 2

Preoperative preparation

The purpose of the anaesthetist's preoperative visit. Preoperative assessment. Preoperative resuscitation. Requirements before transfer to the operating theatre. Preoperative fasting. Premedication. Antibiotic cover. Steroid cover. Other drug therapy. Transportation to theatre. Arrival and waiting in theatre.

The purpose of the anaesthetist's preoperative visit

The purpose of the anaesthetist's visit is to make the acquaintance of the patient, to review the medical history and undertake a physical examination to ensure the patient is fit to have an anaesthetic. The anaesthetist also needs to know what drugs the patient is taking so that dangerous interactions with anaesthetic drugs can be avoided. Preparation for the anaesthetic includes giving an explanation about what will happen, especially if the patient has not had a previous anaesthetic, and generally giving reassurance. To avoid alarming patients when recovering from anaesthesia it is wise to tell them before surgery if you expect them to awaken with any of the following — intravenous lines, pressure monitoring lines, a nasogastric tube, a catheter, chest drains or nasal packs. If the patient is to be electively ventilated postoperatively this should be explained and he or she should be told that a tracheal tube or tracheostomy will be necessary.

When the patient's physical condition and temperament have been assessed appropriate premedication can be ordered. This may vary depending on whether the surgery is major or minor, elective or emergency.

The anaesthetist should also check that blood is cross matched where necessary and that any special investigations have been done.

3

Preoperative assessment

The assessment of fitness for an anaesthetic is simple when a healthy, young person is presenting for elective surgery. When someone has heart or respiratory disease, is on treatment with several drugs and especially if he or she is old there is a greater chance of complications occurring during anaesthesia (i.e. the risk is greater).

Review of the medical history and the physical examination may indicate to the anaesthetist that some modification of the anaesthetic may be necessary. For instance patients with heart disease, particularly fixed cardiac output conditions such as aortic stenosis, should be given myocardial depressant drugs with great care otherwise a disastrous decrease in cardiac output may occur. Patients with asthma should be adequately treated so that they are not wheezing preoperatively, and drugs which cause histamine release and bronchospasm such as morphine and D-tubocurarine should be avoided in the premedication and during anaesthesia. Patients with diabetes should be well controlled, the insulin dose reduced in proportion to the reduction in calorie intake and the timing of surgery should be arranged so that hypoglycaemia does not occur during anaesthesia. Arrangements can also be made to check blood sugar intraoperatively.

If the operation is not urgent and the patient's condition can be improved (e.g. by physiotherapy, antibiotics and stopping smoking in patients with respiratory disease) the operation should be postponed. Patients for elective surgery with an upper respiratory tract infection who have a temperature or a cough should usually be postponed to avoid causing more serious respiratory complications.

If there is some urgency to proceed with surgery then greater risks may be taken although as much should be done to improve the patient's condition as time will permit.

Some people think that anaesthetists are not particularly interested in people as most of their contact is with unconscious patients. This should not be the case as they have to be able to gain rapport with their patients, elucidate any significant medical problems and provide appropriate counselling and reassurance within the space of a relatively short preoperative visit.

The conduct of the preoperative visit with a child will vary with the age of the child. The anaesthetist has to gain rapport and the confidence of the child, and the parents like to be reassured that their child will be cared for sympathetically and competently. Sometimes anxious parents need as much or more reassurance than the child. Relief of this anxiety is important as anxious parents often convey their anxiety to their child.

The anaesthetist will often tell the patient, especially if he is a child, that he is going to put him to sleep for the operation so that he will not feel anything while it is being done. It is always important to tell a child that he will be woken up at the end of the operation, otherwise he may think that he is like a dog or cat being taken away to be put to sleep for ever. Depending on how much the child understands he may be told something about how he will be put to sleep and how he will feel afterwards, and that a short time will be spent in the recovery room before returning to the ward. He should also be told the people working in the theatre will be dressed differently, and may not be recognized easily because they will be wearing masks and caps. Many anaesthetists remove their masks so that the patient can see their face.

Children may be prepared before admission by reading books about hospital, by showing a film or a tape-slide programme about the procedure which occurs when they are admitted and the places they will be taken to in the ward and theatre areas.

Preoperative resuscitation

Patients may have been ill for some time and, particularly before emergency surgery, may need resuscitation. They may be hypovolaemic due to haemorrhage or dehydration, the latter from vomiting, diarrhoea, loss of fluid into the gut or peritoneal cavity or lack of fluid intake. Any deficiency should be corrected before anaesthesia if possible, otherwise the depressant effect of anaesthetic drugs on the heart and brain may be exaggerated and the dose used for a healthy person becomes an overdose.

The fluids used in resuscitation will depend on the type of loss. Patients who have been vomiting will have lost hydrochloric acid from the stomach, as well as some potassium, so will require isotonic saline (0.9%) with potassium chloride supplements.

Losses into the peritoneal cavity may contain much protein. If the i.v. solution does not contain protein or an osmotically active substance such as dextran, much will be lost from the circulation due to a lack of osmotically active particles which hold the fluid in the circulation (Fig. 2.1). Blood loss can be treated initially with a plasma volume expander (stable plasma protein solution, dextran or Haemaccel) or a balanced electrolyte solution such as Hartmann's solution. When blood loss

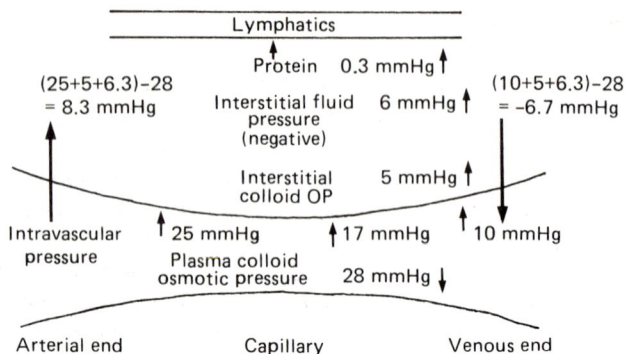

Fig. 2.1 The opposing pressures which determine fluid shifts between capillaries and the surrounding tissues.

exceeds 15–20% of the blood volume, blood is usually transfused. Normal blood volume is about 70 ml/kg and is slightly more in infants, 80 ml/kg.

The anaesthetist will not usually accept a patient for anaesthesia until resuscitation is complete unless there is an acute surgical reason to proceed, such as major uncontrolled bleeding where blood is being lost faster than the transfusion is running in. It is worth remembering that hypovolaemic, dehydrated or uraemic patients may be confused and irrational, and that their language and behaviour may not be characteristic of their normal personality. They call for extra understanding and compassionate care.

Preoperative investigations

Usually some basic information such as temperature, pulse, blood pressure and respiratory rate as well as haemoglobin and urinalysis is obtained before anaesthesia. Other laboratory information such as electrolytes, acid base measurements, blood examination and X-rays may also be requested. These are usually done to confirm the diagnosis and to ensure that the patient is in a satisfactory condition to undergo anaesthesia and surgery. Blood should be cross matched if significant losses at surgery are expected.

Preoperative fasting

Normally patients are fasted for several hours before a general anaesthetic. The reason for this is to allow the stomach to empty so that during induction of anaesthesia vomiting followed by aspiration of stomach contents will not occur. This may result in airway obstruction or, if very acid, acute pulmonary oedema may occur (Mendelson's syndrome). The time taken for the stomach to empty varies but usually 4-6 hours is sufficient. Patients who have been injured or who are very apprehensive may have delayed emptying due to the stress response stimulating the sympathetic nervous system. This inhibits peristalsis. Gastric emptying is also delayed following the administration of narcotic analgesics such as morphine.

At least 6 hours fasting is desirable after solid food and 4 hours after liquids. Most people easily tolerate a fast of this length or longer but infants who have a high metabolic rate and less metabolic reserve should be starved for the shorter period — usually 4 hours after milk and 2–3 hours after clear fluids.

When the operation is urgent then the added risk of a full stomach has to be accepted and the necessary precautions taken (e.g. cricoid pressure, see Chapter 7). Antacids may be given, especially in obstetrics where they reduce the acidity and thereby decrease the chance of potentially lethal acid aspiration which is a particular hazard of anaesthesia in these patients.

Premedication

Premedication is usually ordered. If the patient is very anxious a tranquillizer or hypnotic may be ordered for the night before to help the patient to have a good night's sleep.

The timing of the premedication will depend on the drugs used and the route by which they are given. A drug given orally or rectally is usually administered at least 2 hours before, while intramuscular injections are usually given 1–1.25 hours before.

The drugs are used as follows:

1 To allay anxiety (tranquillizers such as diazepam or promethazine).
2 Sometimes to provide analgesia to relieve preoperative pain or to provide some of the analgesia during the operation (morphine, papaveretum (omnopon), pethidine).

3 To dry secretions in the mouth and respiratory tract and to block vagal reflexes (atropine and hyoscine).

Some of these drugs have more than one use. For instance, morphine and papaveretum also produce some euphoria which reduces apprehension, while hyoscine acts centrally on the brain to produce some sedation and amnesia and suppress vomiting. Thus the combination of intramuscular papaveretum and hyoscine provides a well sedated, tranquil patient who may not remember much of the visit to the operating theatre afterwards. The combination of pethidine, promethazine and atropine is often used for asthmatics because morphine and papaveretum cause histamine release which can precipitate bronchospasm. The problem with the former combination is that it requires two injections which most patients do not relish.

Many anaesthetists prefer to avoid premedication which requires an injection in children. In some places no premedication is used, the reassurance of the child being dependent on experienced and sympathetic staff who stay with the child during the preoperative period. Oral premedication, usually a tranquillizer such as promethazine (Phenergan), trimeprazine (Vallergan), diazepam (valium), lorazepam or chlorpromazine (Largactil) can be given as a suspension. These are well absorbed if given 2 hours before operation and usually provide a reasonably tranquil patient without the need for an injection but recovery following anaesthesia may be delayed especially with trimeprazine. Small infants are often not premedicated and narcotics are not usually used under 6 months of age.

Care must be taken to ensure that the patient receives the correct dose of drug. Doses are more often related to weight in children. The commonest sources of error are (a) the incorrect weight being recorded on the chart so that the calculated dose is too large or too small, (b) an incorrect dose is ordered and (c) an error in the calculation of how much of an ampoule is to be given. The calculation and amount of drug drawn up in the syringe is always checked by a registered nurse to avoid the latter source of error. The hazard is greatest when an excessive dose of a respiratory depressant drug is given (e.g. morphine, pethidine).

When intramuscular premedication is given the nurse's attitude and technique are important, especially after the injection when the nurse should settle the patient comfortably. A firm but kindly approach is desirable.

It must be stressed again that the sympathetic and considerate handling of the patient plays a very important part in the preoperative preparation of the patient. This cannot be replaced by drugs alone.

Antibiotic cover

Patients who have valvular or congenital heart disease or have had cardiac surgery usually have an antibiotic cover which may be given with the premedication, especially when dental or other oral procedures are to be performed which may result in a bacteraemia. Subacute bacterial endocarditis may follow if an antibiotic cover is not given.

Steroid cover

Hydrocortisone may be given with the premedication to patients on steroid treatment. Long term steroid treatment, especially when high doses are used, suppresses the adrenal cortex so that the secretion of cortisol in response to stress is reduced. This can result in hypotension when anaesthesia is induced. Extra preoperative steroids help to prevent this complication.

Other drug therapy

Some patients are on long term treatment for conditions such as depression, hypertension, asthma, epilepsy or diabetes. The anaesthetist will have to decide how soon before the operation the last dose of these other drugs should be given. The decisions will depend on the likelihood of complications occurring if they are stopped too soon or on the possibility of adverse interactions occurring between the drug and drugs used during anaesthesia.

Preparation for transfer to the operating theatre

Patients are usually washed or have a bath prior to surgery. A hospital gown is usually worn because it can be easily undone and so that the patient's clothes are not soiled.

Jewellery, hair pins and make-up, including nail polish, should be removed. If patients are allowed to keep their dentures in (especially full dentures) they are less embarrassed, the airway is more easily maintained with a mask and they can still be removed prior to intubation if necessary. The anaesthetist should always enquire about dentures. If dentures are left in a labelled denture container they should accompany the patient to theatre. The patient should empty his or her bladder. Identification bands with the patient's name and unit number are checked. The correct history (with recent temperature, pulse and respiratory rate recordings), drug and fluid order sheets, fluid balance chart and any other relevant papers including a signed consent form for anaesthesia and surgery should accompany the patient. In some hospitals the check list from theatre specifies which of these are required. The rules for the transfer of the patient's X-rays and blood, if ordered, vary in different hospitals but the appropriate arrangements should be made.

Transportation to theatre

The patient should be helped on to the trolley and must be made to feel secure. The trolley sides should be raised or, in their absence, patients should be strapped on to the trolley. In the case of small children, cot sides should be raised to prevent them from rolling off. The patient should be made as comfortable as possible with pillows and adequately covered with blankets for warmth and privacy. (Theatre gowns can be revealing!)

It is advantageous if a nurse who has been looking after the patient accompanies him or her to theatre because of the reassurance gained from a familiar face. This is particularly true in the case of children, the elderly or anyone who is very apprehensive.

The management of children requires special consideration. The personality and attitude of the porters and staff taking patients to theatre can make a difference. Someone who takes an interest in the patient can have a reassuring influence. The timing of separation of children from their parents is worthy of consideration. It is often easiest for the parent and the child if this occurs when the child settles following the onset of the effect of the premedication. Separation at the theatre entrance is undesirable as many children handle one upsetting circumstance at a time but not the combined effect of parental separation and entry to a strange environment.

In some places a parent is allowed to accompany the child to the induction room and remains until the child falls asleep. This has some advantages with small children or where a child has complex congenital anomalies and has had many operations or procedures and is frightened of more, but there are also some problems. It will not be in the child's interest if the anaesthetist does not feel completely at ease having the particular parent present. To succeed the parent must be able to cope with the situation. When it comes to the point some parents become anxious, make their child apprehensive and increase the stress to the anaesthetist at a critical time. The end result can be detrimental to the child. Some children tend to play off the anaesthetist against the parent with distracting results. Some anaesthetists find the presence of a stranger at induction adds unacceptably to an already stressful period of their work. It can be compared to the distraction which would occur if airline pilots or bus drivers were disturbed by passengers.

The presence of parents at induction is easier to handle in small hospitals or units and in some outpatient facilities but in theatre complexes with a large number of patients being operated upon each day the logistics of having extra people gowned and masked may become very time consuming and costly and interfere with the flow of work. It may also require extra staff to look after them.

Ultimately it should be the anaesthetist who decides when parents can be admitted to the induction room. Usually when the child is adequately premedicated and the anaesthetist has developed some rapport with the patient the child copes adequately without a parent being present.

Arrival and waiting in theatre

On arrival in the theatre reception area a check is made to ensure that the correct patient has arrived and that the name tags and documents have the same name and unit number. On rare occasions two patients with the same name are scheduled for different operations. It is very important that the correct chart, X-rays and blood accompany each patient. It is also wise for the anaesthetist or surgeon to check with the patient what operation is to be done and on which side.

Patients should be spoken to, preferably addressed by name, while waiting in the theatre reception area if they are awake. This helps to relieve their anxiety and the sense of loneliness which can develop if they are ignored. The staff must be aware of the presence of patients and not carry on inappropriate conversations within earshot. Patients should not be left unobserved while waiting, should be kept warm and comfortable and if delays occur they should be informed.

The waiting period is much easier for children if there is a kindly person who talks and comforts them and if appropriate reads to them from a book.

CHAPTER 3

Equipment and its cleaning

EQUIPMENT   The anaesthetic machine. Circuits. Warning devices. Scavenging. Ventilators. Masks. Airways. Head harness. Endotracheal tubes. Laryngoscopes. Introducer. Suction. Intravenous needles and cannulae. Regional anaesthetic equipment. Special trays.
CLEANING   Cleanliness. Decontamination. Methods of sterilization. Methods of disinfection. Management of specific items of equipment. Infected cases.

Equipment

The anaesthetic machine

Anaesthetic machines (Fig. 3.1) are designed to supply oxygen and the anaesthetic gases and vapours which are inhaled by the patient during anaesthesia. They also provide some space for drugs, syringes and equipment such as laryngoscopes and monitoring equipment.

The gas supply may be from cylinders on the machine or from a bulk supply carried through a hose from the wall to the machine. It should not be possible to interchange the oxygen and nitrous oxide connections. A pin index system on the cylinders prevents a cylinder being attached to the wrong gas line and different bayonet fittings prevent inappropriate connections of the gas hose pipeline.

The gases are passed through flowmeters so that gas flows can be measured and the concentrations of oxygen and nitrous oxide administered can be accurately controlled. The commonest variety of flowmeter is a rotameter (Fig. 3.2) which has a gradually widening glass tube with a spinning bobbin which rises higher as the gas flow increases. The flow is indicated on a graduated scale on the tube.

The gases may then be passed through a vaporizer which contains a liquid anaesthetic such as halothane (Fluothane), enflurane (Ethrane) or methoxyflurane (Penthrane). The simplest form or vaporizer is the

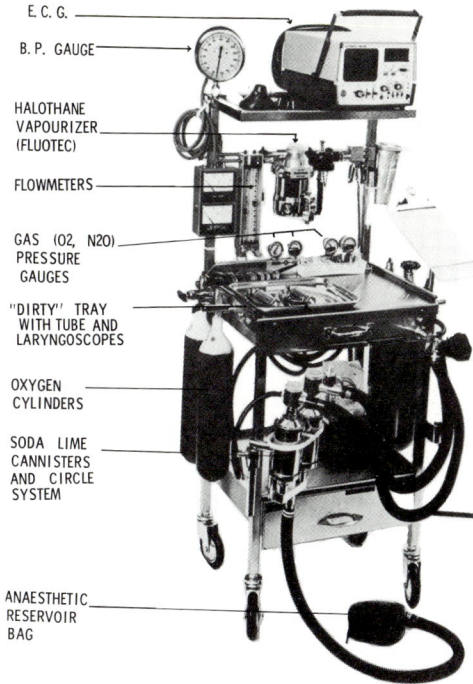

E. C. G.

B. P. GAUGE

HALOTHANE
VAPOURIZER
(FLUOTEC)

FLOWMETERS

GAS (02, N2O)
PRESSURE
GAUGES

"DIRTY" TRAY
WITH TUBE AND
LARYNGOSCOPES

OXYGEN
CYLINDERS

SODA LIME
CANNISTERS
AND CIRCLE
SYSTEM

ANAESTHETIC
RESERVOIR
BAG

Fig. 3.1   A commonly used 'Boyles' type anaesthetic machine showing important components.

Boyle bottle (Fig. 3.3) originally used for ether. The gas is passed over the liquid picking up anaesthetic in the vapour phase as it goes and if a higher concentration is desired the gas may be bubbled through the liquid. With the advent of more potent anaesthetics, such as halothane, more complex vaporizers such as the Fluotec were developed. These deliver an accurate concentration under varying conditions of temperature and gas flow.

Before an anaesthetic is begun the machine should be checked to ensure that there is an adequate supply of gases (indicated on the gauges) and that the vaporizers contain the appropriate anaesthetic agent. Special filling attachments are now available, each specific for one anaesthetic agent and its vaporizer. If halothane could be put in a Pentec vaporizer a concentration of 30% could be achieved in the circuit. This would quickly overdose the patient with a fatal result. The difference is that in the Fluotec vaporizer most of the carrier gas bypasses the vapor-

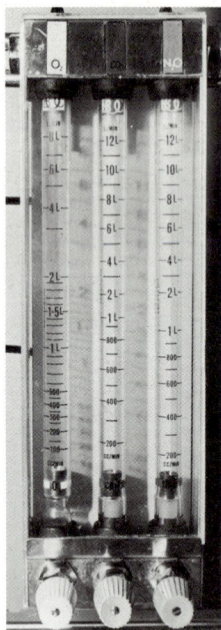

Fig. 3.2 Flowmeters graduated for specific gases. The tube gradually widens from bottom to top allowing increasing flow rates of gas to flow past the bobbin which should rotate during normal function.

izing chamber. Halothane boils at 50.2°C and has a vapour pressure at 20°C of 240 mmHg which is much higher than that required for anaesthesia. Methoxyflurane (Penthrane) boils at 104°C and has a vapour pressure at 20°C of 23 mmHg. The maximum concentration of methoxyflurane at 20°C is 3% (23/760 × 100) but for halothane it is 28% (240/760 × 100).

Circuits

The available circuits can be classified as (a) rebreathing with carbon dioxide absorption, (b) partial rebreathing, which have been subdivided into the Mapleson A to E systems and (c) non rebreathing.

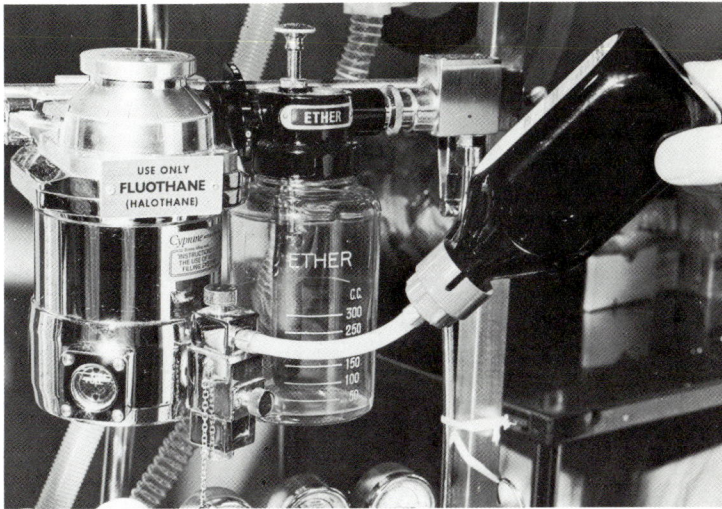

Fig. 3.3 A Mark 3 Fluotec vaporizer being filled via a filler which will only fit this vaporizer and the halothane bottle. Next to it is the Boyle bottle vaporizer.

(a) *Rebreathing circuits with carbon dioxide absorption*

These include the widely used circle system (Fig. 3.1) in which the gas enters the circuit from the machine and can be reused because the patient's exhaled carbon dioxide is absorbed by soda lime contained in the canisters. Economy and minimal pollution can be achieved if very low gas flows are used.

It is important with low flows to ensure that there is an adequate flow of oxygen from the machine to prevent the patient becoming hypoxic, because oxygen will be continually removed from the circuit by the patient. Basal oxygen requirement is about 250 ml/minute. Many anaesthetic machines now incorporate an oxygen analyser with a low level alarm in the circuit to monitor the oxygen concentration of the gas which the patient is breathing. When higher gas flows are used the excess gas escapes from an exhale valve on the expiratory limb.

The other circuit with carbon dioxide absorption depends on the patient breathing to and fro into a Waters' canister containing soda lime (Fig. 3.4). This is now rarely used but as the Waters' canister can be

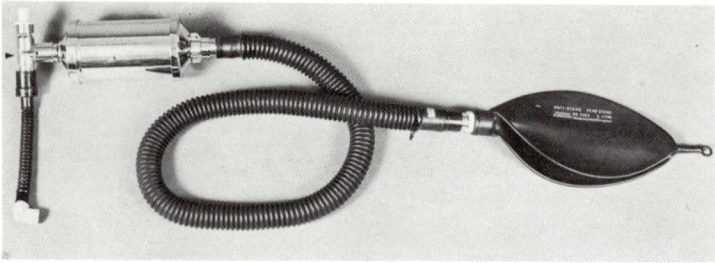

Fig. 3.4 The Waters' canister is placed near the endotracheal tube attachment and expiratory valve. The patient can rebreathe into the canister when carbon dioxide is absorbed. The fresh gas requirements are thus reduced and the system is less bulky and more easily sterilized than the circle.

autoclaved it can be used in patients with respiratory infections such as tuberculosis where sterilization of equipment is difficult.

(b) *Partial rebreathing circuits*

These may take several forms but basically include an expiratory valve, a reservoir bag, a variable length of tubing and a fresh gas inlet. Figure 3.5 illustrates the various arrangements as classified by Mapleson. When the patient is breathing spontaneously (on his own without assistance) (a) is the best circuit. The fresh gas flow needed to ensure that carbon dioxide

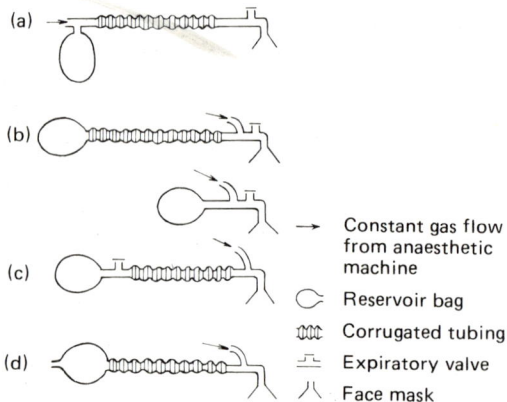

Fig. 3.5 Classification of partial rebreathing circuits.

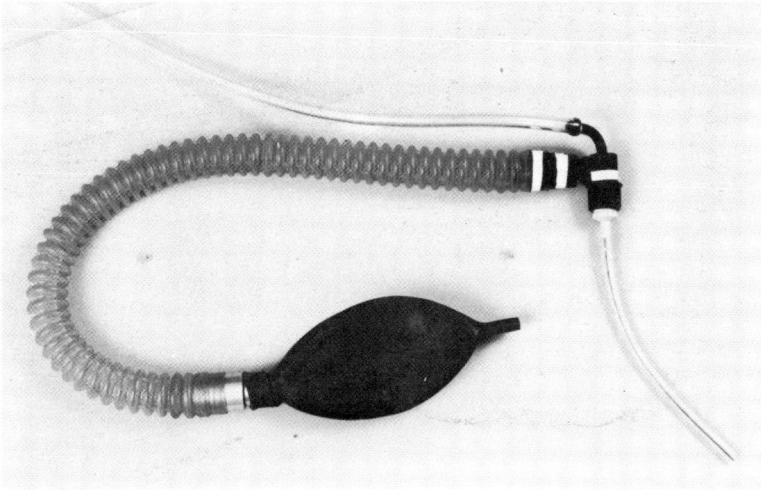

Fig. 3.6 A 'Jackson Rees' modification of the Ayres T piece circuit showing the line bringing fresh gases from the machine (top), a T piece connection with an endotracheal tube and the expiratory limb with a bag on the end.

expired by the patient is not rebreathed, thereby causing a rise in P_{CO_2} (see Chapter 4) is 0.7 of the minute volume (tidal volume × respiratory rate). During controlled ventilation circuit (d) is the most efficient. The T-piece with the bag on the end of the expiratory limb and the Bain circuits which are described below are in this category.

In paediatric anaesthesia the T-piece system, which may have a bag on the expiratory limb (Fig. 3.6), is commonly used. An adequate fresh gas flow from the machine is required to ensure elimination of carbon dioxide and the expiratory limb must have a volume exceeding tidal volume to ensure that the anaesthetic gases are not diluted by air during inspiration. The advantages of the circuit are the low resistance because there are no valves, its low dead space (see The Anaesthetic Machine above) and its simplicity.

When the Jackson Rees modification of the T-piece with an open ended bag on the end of the expiratory limb is used in controlled ventilation the open end is closed so that the bag fills, the bag is then compressed thus inflating the patient and then the open end is released to allow expiration to occur (Fig. 3.7). When a mechanical ventilator is attached to the expiratory limb the latter must have a greater volume

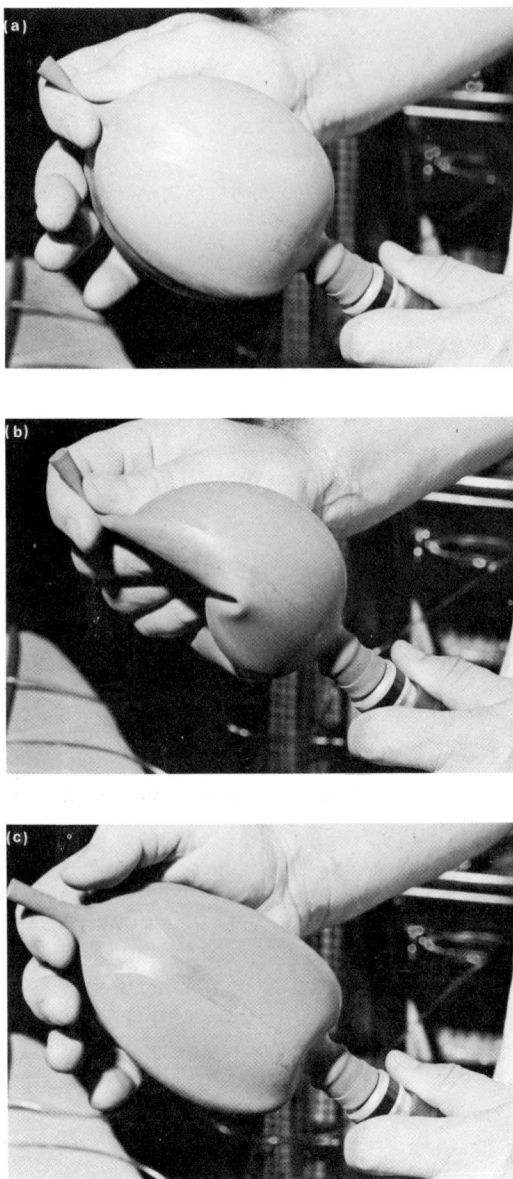

Fig. 3.7   Ventilation with an open ended bag using one hand. (a) The open tail is occluded so that the bag fills. (b) The bag is then compressed thus inflating the patient. (c) The tail of the bag is released to allow expiration.

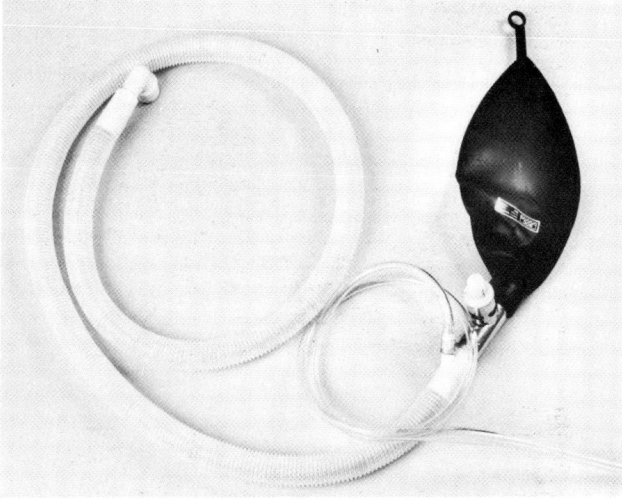

Fig. 3.8 A Bain circuit with the fresh gas line entering the corrugated tubing near the bag. The fresh gas line passes along to the distal connection for mask or tube (upper left). The expired gas then returns along the corrugated tube outside the fresh gas line to the expiratory valve and reservoir bag. In this system the fresh gas is partly warmed by the expired gas before reaching the patient.

than the tidal volume delivered, otherwise the gas delivered from the ventilator will dilute the anaesthetic.

The Bain circuit (Fig. 3.8) has the fresh gas flow line running down the inside of the expiratory limb. It can be used as a modified T-piece with an open ended bag or as a Mapleson D circuit with a closed bag and an expiratory valve.

The circle system can be used without soda lime absorbers but the gas flow required to maintain carbon dioxide homeostasis is higher. With this system and with the T-piece and Bain circuits adjustments to fresh gas flow can be used to set the $P\text{CO}_2$ level when controlled ventilation is used. The usual range to maintain a $P\text{CO}_2$ at or slightly below 40 mmHg is 70–100 ml/kg or, for the T-piece in children, the square root of body weight × 0.8 l/minute.

(c) *Non rebreathing circuits*
These employ a one way valve such as the Lewis Leigh, Stephen Slater or Ruben valves. They allow fresh gas to enter the patient from the

machine in inspiration. In expiration the expired gas closes the valve temporarily stopping fresh gas inflow while the patient expires to the atmosphere. These valves were popular in North America but are not widely used now.

The circle system conserves some of the exhaled water vapour so that some humidification of the inspired gases occurs. In the T-piece system gases delivered to the patient will be dry unless a humidifier is placed in the gas line before delivery to the patient. This is now commonly done especially in infant anaesthesia so that the gases can be warmed and humidified. This reduces heat loss and prevents water loss from the respiratory tract with drying of the respiratory epithelium. Possible decrease in ciliary activity resulting in accumulation of mucus in peripheral airways is thus prevented. The details of checking the circuit are discussed in Chapter 6.

Warning devices

Other additional devices may be added to the machine mostly aimed to increase safety. An oxygen alarm (e.g. Howeson, Bosun) which whistles when the oxygen supply runs out is usually present. A pressure gauge in the circuit will show if excessively high pressures are developing or that the pressure has dropped due to disconnection in the circuit or failure of the gas supply. There are usually gauges to indicate the gas pressures in the cylinders so that the anaesthetist has some warning that a cylinder is nearly empty. Oxygen in cylinders is a compressed gas and the pressure will fall steadily as the gas is used. Nitrous oxide, on the other hand, is a liquid under pressure with a gas phase above the liquid. The pressure recorded is the gas pressure and it will remain constant until all the liquid has vaporized and then the pressure will fall rapidly.

Additional devices which may be used are as follows:
1 An oxygen analyser to measure the oxygen concentration.
2 A capnograph which measures carbon dioxide concentration. End expired carbon dioxide will rise if ventilation is inadequate and can signify a gas leak from the circuit or it may fall due to hyperventilation. A sudden decrease can signify air embolism which is an uncommon complication most likely to occur in neurosurgery when air enters an open vein.
3 A respirometer may be included to measure tidal volume.
4 Disconnection alarm.

Scavenging

Various methods of collecting.exhaled gases are now in common use in an effort to reduce the pollution of the operating theatres. The gases are usually discarded through the ventilation system or via the suction and eliminated outside to the atmosphere.

Ventilators

When patients are paralysed with muscle relaxants ventilation must be maintained by intermittent squeezing of the anaesthetic reservoir bag by hand or by the use of a mechanical ventilator.

There are many ventilators available but detailed description of them is beyond the scope of this book. Those used in the operating theatre can generally be simpler than the more sophisticated ventilators used in intensive care units but there are many used in both situations. Ventilators may be powered by gas or electricity. High pressure gas driven ventilators are usually powered by pipeline oxygen and low pressure-gas-driven ventilators by the anaesthetic gases from a Boyle's Machine.

The complete respiratory cycle of a ventilator may be divided into four phases: (a) inspiration, (b) switching from inspiration to expiration, (c) expiration and (d) switching from expiration to inspiration. Four functions, which are interrelated, are involved in controlling these phases. They are volume, pressure, flow and time.

$$Flow = volume/time.$$

$$Pressure = flow \times resistance \text{ (cf. Ohms Law)}.$$

Resistance depends on airways resistance and to a lesser extent on compliance of the lung and iung volume (see Respiratory System, Chapter 4).

The variations in types of ventilators depends on the functions used in the different phases. Normally two of these determine the volume delivered in inspiration. For instance a flow generator ventilator will deliver a volume which depends on the fresh gas flow rate and the time taken for the inspiratory phase. The gas flow pattern into the lung is shown in Fig. 3.9a which differs from that delivered by a pressure generator (Fig. 3.9b) which can produce more variation. One function is

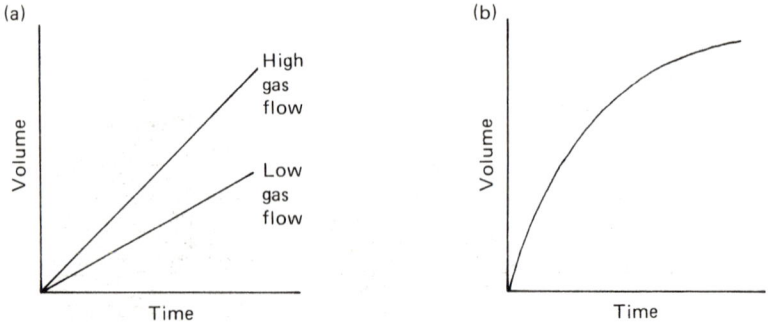

Fig. 3.9 The different patterns of gas flow into the lungs with (a) flow and (b) pressure generator ventilators. The volume delivered by a flow generator in a given time is dependent on the fresh gas flow from the machine, whereas with a pressure generator the volume increases rapidly at first and then at a gradually decreasing rate as the pressure in the lung rises.

normally used to switch the ventilator from inspiration to expiration. This usually occurs when a set volume has been delivered, the preset pressure has been reached or a given time has elapsed. Expiration (phase 3) and the change to inspiration (phase 4) are usually dependent on time (time cycled).

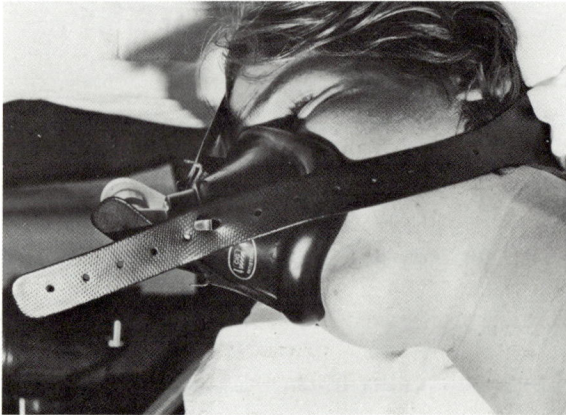

Fig. 3.10 The anaesthetic can be delivered via a face mask. It is important to ensure that the jaw is held so that the tongue does not fall back and obstruct the pharyngeal airway. This mask is held in place with a head harness.

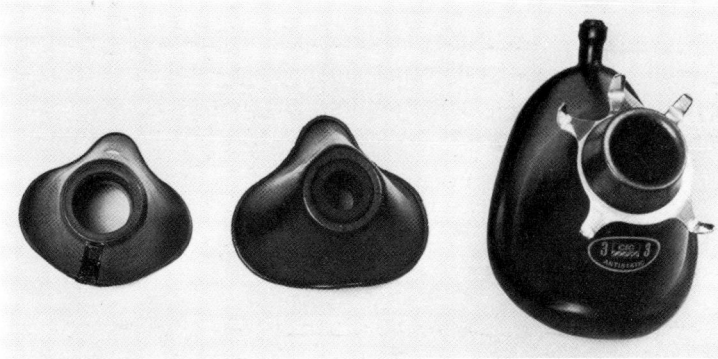

Fig. 3.11 Face masks. (Right) Adult mask with an inflatable cushion to facilitate fitting the face. The plug should be removed before autoclaving. The clips are for attaching a head harness. (Centre and left) Two sizes of smaller Rendell Baker masks for infants or children. These are specially constructed to have a small dead space and do not have a cushioned rim.

Some ventilators have the additional ability to subject the airway to a small positive or negative pressure during phase 3 (expiration). Ventilators used in the operating theatre often compress a bag or bellows which replaces the anaesthetic reservoir bag.

Masks

Oxygen and anaesthetic gases can be delivered to the patient via a face mask (Fig. 3.10). These come in various sizes (Fig. 3.11). Adult masks usually have a circumferential inflatable cushion to allow a closer fit on to the face.

Small masks for children (Rendell Baker-Soucek) are specially designed so that the volume of the space between the face and mask is minimized. This volume contributes to the anaesthetic dead space. Dead space is that part of the breath (tidal volume) which does not reach the alveoli for gas exchange to take place (see Chapter 4). It is important in infants and small children, who have small dead spaces and tidal volumes, to keep the mask dead space to a minimum so that a significant decrease in alveolar ventilation with carbon dioxide retention is avoided.

Airways

When a mask is used it may be difficult to maintain an airway which allows the patient to breath easily. An oropharyngeal airway (Fig. 3.12) can be inserted in the mouth to ensure a free air flow. These often have a metal insert so that when the teeth are clenched the airway is not occluded.

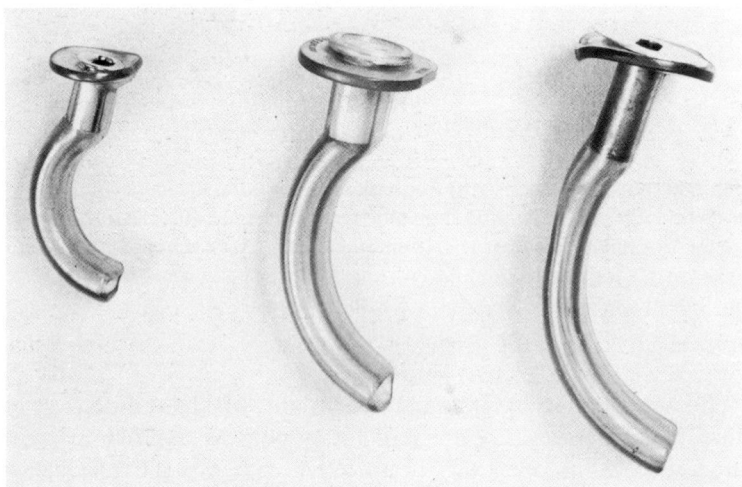

Fig. 3.12   Guedel airways are used to ensure an adequate oral airway. They have a metal or firm plastic insert to prevent the teeth compressing the lumen and causing obstruction. There are several sizes to cater for different sizes of patients.

Head harness

A head harness is sometimes used to hold the mask in place when the patient is breathing spontaneously (Fig. 3.10). This frees the anaesthetist's hand to do other things.

Endotracheal tubes

A variety of endotracheal tubes are available. Formerly red rubber tubes were used but now the tubes are mostly made of polyvinylchloride (PVC) or silastic. These are usually sold as disposable items but some can be resterilized satisfactorily. High temperature autoclaving usually softens

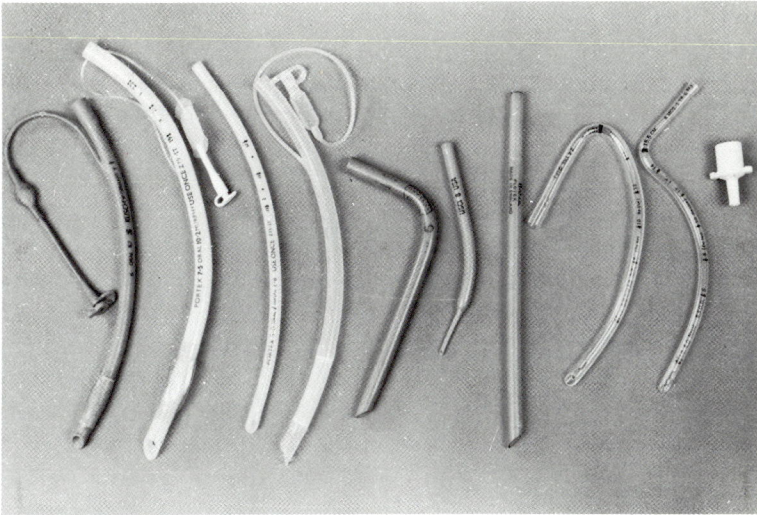

Fig. 3.13 Endotracheal tubes (from left to right). Cuffed red rubber Magill, cuffed and uncuffed PVC, cuffed silastic, Oxford, Cole with narrow terminal segment, and armoured latex which has a spiral wire in the wall to prevent kinking, oral RAE, nasal RAE tubes and a 15 mm plastic connector.

and may distort the PVC tubes making them unsuitable for reuse. Autoclaving at 120°C for longer periods is as effective and is less damaging to the tube making limited reuse feasible. Gamma radiation causes hardening of some plastics after a few exposures. Various types of tubes are shown in Fig. 3.13.

Some tubes are made especially for nasal intubation. These have a rounder, shorter bevel so that they are less likely to gouge into the nasopharyngeal tissues. The RAE nasal tube is preformed so that it turns up over the forehead and thus keeps out of the surgeon's way for procedures around the neck and mouth.

Usually uncuffed tubes are used for patients under 12 years because the narrowest part of the larynx before puberty is the cricoid ring which is circular. After puberty the vocal cord region, which is not circular, becomes the narrowest part. The use of cuffs in small airways requires the use of a smaller tube size resulting in greater airways resistance.

An adult male usually will take a 9 mm cuffed tube and an adult female an 8 mm cuffed tube. The cuff should be inflated to just occlude the leak when positive pressure is applied. In children the size of tube used is approximately age/4 + 4 mm (internal diameter) while neonates usually take a 3.0 mm and infants a 3.5 mm tube. A choice of sizes, the expected size and one larger and one smaller, are usually prepared for paediatric anaesthesia so that if the expected size is too large or too small the next size is readily available to try. The correct size is one which just

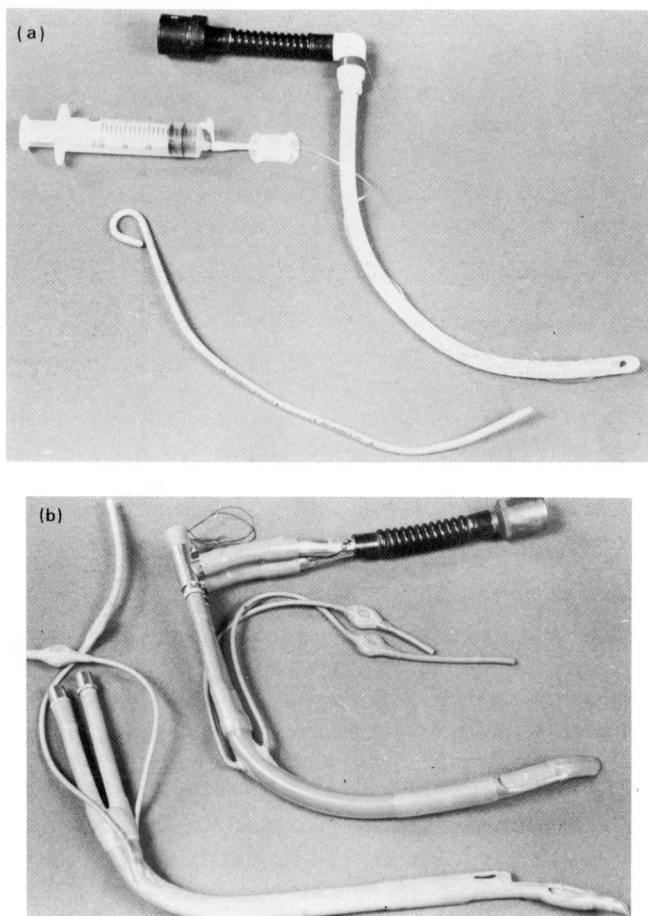

Fig. 3.14 Attachments to connect endotracheal tubes to the circle system used for adults and older children. (a) PVC tube (top) with cuff inflated and connections to the anaesthetic circuit and a stylet (bottom) which can be inserted through the tube to provide curvature during insertion into the trachea. (b) Left Robertshaw double lumen tube with double connector and attachment to circuit (top) and Bryce Smith double lumen with right endo-bronchial tube (bottom). Both have a tracheal (T) and bronchial (B) cuff.

allows a small leak. If the leak is too great very high gas flows are required and it may be difficult to adequately ventilate the patient. If there is no leak pressure on the mucosa may lead to postoperative laryngeal oedema which may narrow the airway and cause stridor.

When an endotracheal tube is inserted, usually through the mouth but occasionally through the nose, the correct connectors between the tube and the remainder of the circuit must be available before anaesthesia is commenced (Figs. 3.14 and 3.15).

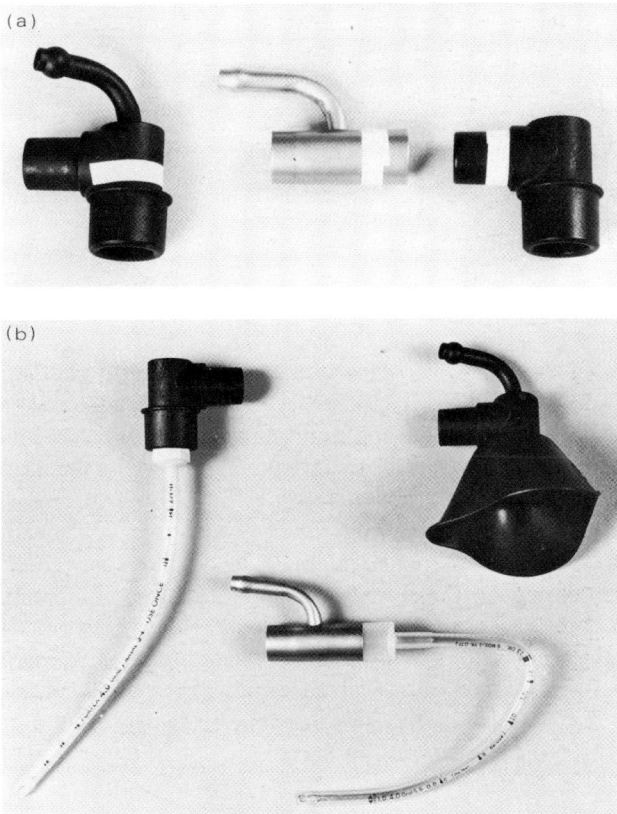

Fig. 3.15   (a) Three useful 15/22 mm paediatric connections. (Right) Gas inlet, expiratory connection and 15 mm internal opening for endotracheal tube and 22 mm external diameter to fit into a face mask. (Centre) Fresh gas inlet port with 15 mm external and 15 mm internal fittings. The latter can connect to an endotracheal tube or the right angled attachment shown (left). (b) Paediatric connections with mask or endotracheal tubes attached.

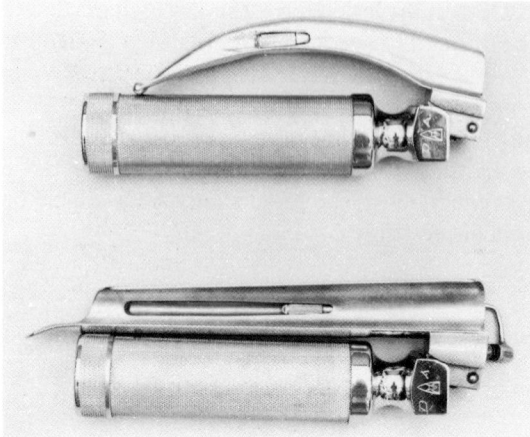

Fig. 3.16 Laryngoscopes, with Macintosh blade (above) and Magill straight blade (below).

Laryngoscopes

Laryngoscopes are used to view the larynx during intubation of the trachea and for inspection of the pharynx during suction. They usually have a battery in the handle and a bulb situated on the blade. It is useful in children with small mouths to have the light near the tip of the blade so that the maximum intensity of light is achieved inside the mouth. The blades may be straight (e.g. Magill) or curved (e.g. Macintosh) (Fig. 3.16). In small children small straight blades are often used (Fig. 3.17a), while in obstetrics the Kennell blade facilitates intubation (Fig. 3.17b).

The laryngoscope is held in the left hand during intubation. The mouth is opened and the blade advanced down the right hand side of the mouth. There is a bar on the left side of the blade to prevent the tongue from obstructing the view of the larynx.

Introducer

Occasionally when intubation is difficult a pliable introducer is lubricated and passed through the lumen of the tube and curved so that the tip of the tube can be directed through the larynx (Fig. 3.13 right hand tube). Alternatively a Magill forceps can be used (Fig. 3.18).

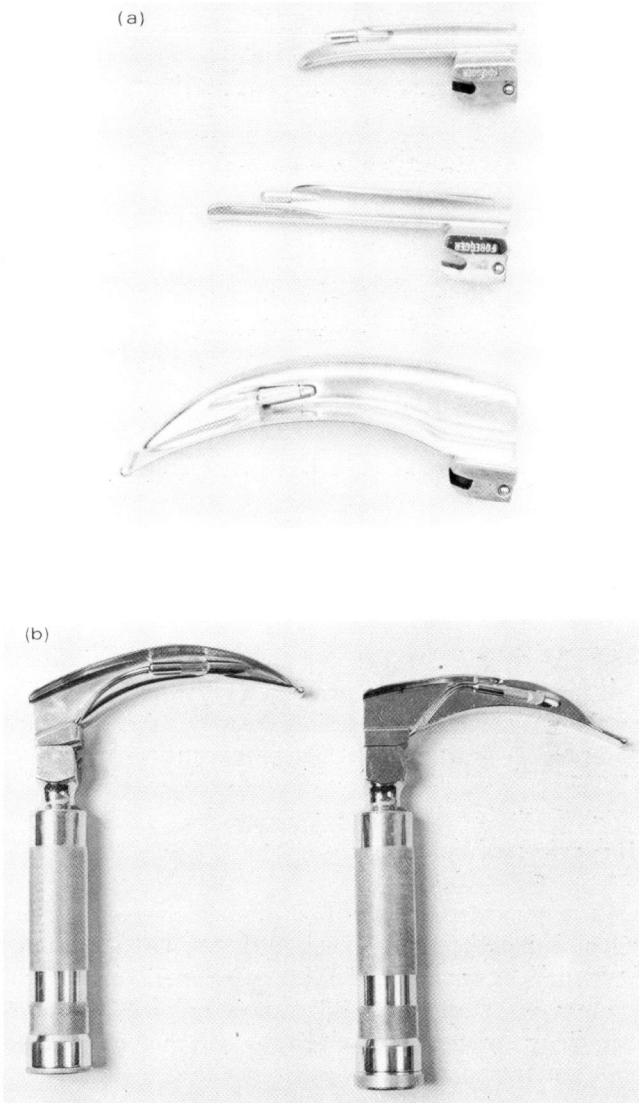

Fig. 3.17 (a) Laryngoscope blades (top) newborn size, (middle) infant and small child size, (bottom) adult Macintosh blade useful for adults and older children. Note that the bulbs are near the tip which makes them suitable for small children because the light is concentrated within the mouth (cf. Fig. 3.8 Magill blade). (b) Kennell blade (left) which is useful in obstetric anaesthesia because the angle between the blade and handle is increased.

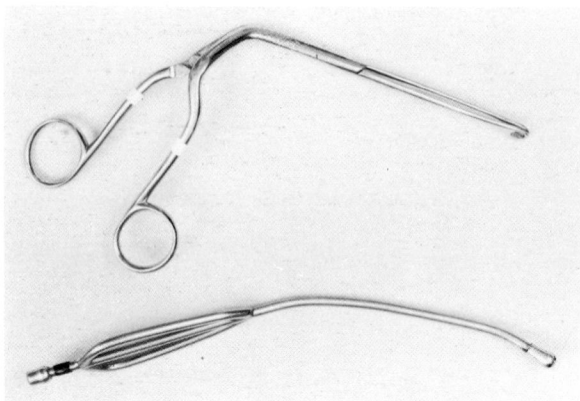

Fig. 3.18   Magill forceps (top). These are used to guide endotracheal tubes into the larynx, to insert throat packs and to grasp objects in the pharynx. Yankauer sucker (below) is a curved metal sucker for suctioning the pharynx and mouth. Before use the tip must be checked to see that it is firmly screwed on.

Suction

A working sucker (Fig. 3.18) should always be available especially at induction and the conclusion of anaesthesia. Usually a central hospital system with wall outlets in all operating theatres, anaesthetic rooms and the recovery room provides the negative pressure for suction.

Intravenous needles and cannulae

Access to a vein for administration of the induction agent and for giving fluids, blood and drugs during anaesthesia is required for most anaesthetics nowadays. A winged needle such as a Butterfly needle will often suffice but for major surgery an intravenous cannula is more reliable. There are many varieties of these and the one chosen will depend on availability and the anaesthetist's preference (Fig. 3.19).

Regional anaesthetic equipment

Prepacked sterile trays, containing standard equipment, may be used for most regional blocks. A bowl, for the local anaesthetic solution, forceps, swabs, two large bore drawing up needles, appropriate syringes (e.g.

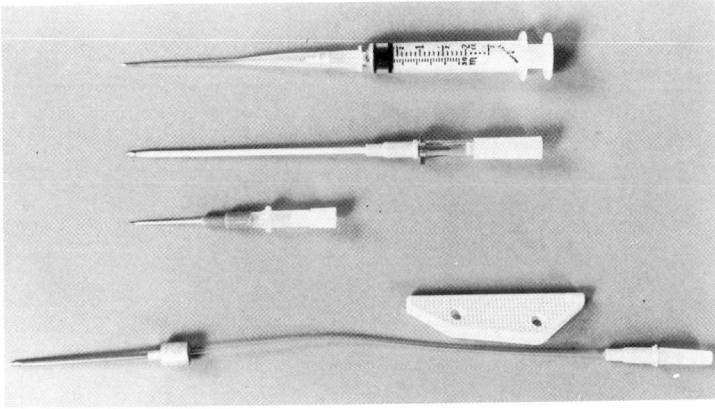

Fig. 3.19 Intravenous cannulae. In the right-hand three the needle is inside the cannula whereas in the left-hand one the cannula is passed through a larger needle. The protective clip is placed over the needle to prevent it from cutting the cannula.

10 ml and 2 ml) and sterile towels are required. If local anaesthetic solution is to be injected intrathecally (spinal anaesthesia) the ampoule or vial should also be included in the sterile pack. Some hospitals may also include Tuohy needles (for epidural anaesthesia) and spinal needles

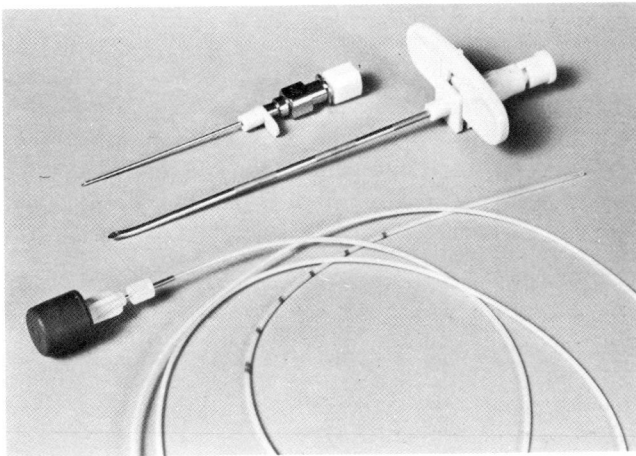

Fig. 3.20 A spinal needle with stillette (top). A Tuohy epidural needle through which a catheter can be passed and directed (middle). An epidural catheter (bottom).

(Fig. 3.20) in their sterile packs. Swabs soaked with antiseptic solution should be stored separately in a plastic container thereby avoiding contamination of the local anaesthetic solution or their accidental interposition when two bowls are used for the local anaesthetic and the antiseptic solution.

Additional equipment which may be added to the pack when it is opened will vary according to the block to be performed. It includes Tuohy needles, epidural catheters, spinal needles, special nerve block needles, plastic disposable syringes and local anaesthetic solution.

Toxic reactions to local anaesthetic agents may occur if the local anaesthetic is inadvertently given intravenously. The major manifestations of toxicity are convulsions, loss of consciousness and, at higher blood levels, cardiovascular depression. Regional blocks should therefore not be undertaken without (a) intravenous access, (b) equipment for ventilation with oxygen, (c) suction and (d) drugs and fluid for resuscitation.

Special trays

A variety of sterilized trays are available in many hospitals for specific procedures. Sometimes when cannulating a vein or artery it is useful to have a small tray with sterile gauze, cotton wool, scissors, a small pair of artery forceps, a pair of dissecting forceps, a scalpel for cutting down on the vessel if necessary and possibly a small bowl for antiseptic solution.

Patients undergoing cardiac or neurosurgery or some other major surgery may require a urinary catheter to be passed. A tray with sterile towels, swabs, a bowl for antiseptic solution, a swab holder, a pair of forceps and a syringe is used. A separately packaged sterile catheter and gloves are also needed.

Cleaning

Cleanliness

Infections may be transmitted to patients by dirty hands contaminating equipment or by organisms collecting on anaesthetic equipment, particularly those parts of the breathing circuit nearest the patient. The potential for transmission of organisms can be reduced by clean habits and by appropriate cleaning and disinfection or sterilization of equipment.

There should be a designated area on the anaesthetic machine and/or trolley for dirty equipment. Often this is put on a towel but a metal tray, bowl or other container which can be washed between cases is preferable because contamination of the underlying surface is avoided and laundry costs are eliminated. Figure 3.1 shows such a 'dirty' tray on the top of the anaesthetic machine and a milk shake container on the right hand upright for discarded items. Syringes and needles can be kept separate by placing them either on a foil tray, which can be autoclaved, or on a sterile towel.

Washing hands between cases is an important step in reducing contamination of equipment and transmission of microorganisms to patients.

Decontamination

The first step in cleaning is to wash reusable equipment such as masks, airways and endotracheal tubes ensuring that any mucus or potentially infected debris is removed. This may require scrubbing the inside with a bottle brush using soap and water. Effective cleaning reduces the number of microorganisms present and provides a smooth clean surface which is more accessible to decontaminating agents. Removal of mucus and debris from endotracheal tubes ensures that they are not obstructed.

Equipment may then be sterilized, disinfected or pasteurized. *Sterilization* is a process that is intended to kill or remove *all* living organisms, including resistant bacterial spores. *Disinfection* is a process that is intended to kill or remove disease producing microorganisms (pathogens) but not eliminate all bacterial spores. *Pasteurization* is a process of disinfection by hot water or steam at a temperature between 65°C and 100°C.

Methods of sterilization

(a) *Heat*
High temperature sterilizers with steam: the temperatures required vary from 121°C to 134°C. The higher the temperature and the lower the

pressure the shorter the period required. The units operate at 132°C for 3 minutes (for unwrapped articles) at 121°C for 30 minutes or at 132–134°C for 6 minutes in prevacuum sterilizers (wrapped articles). Dry heat is not used for sterilizing anaesthetic equipment.

(b) *Ethylene oxide*
This is suitable for heat sensitive materials but sufficient time must elapse for removal of the gas after treatment. Tissue damage can occur from exposure to ethylene oxide. For this reason it is better not to use it for breathing apparatus so that the potential hazard of accidental damage due to inadequate venting of the ethylene oxide is avoided.

(c) *Gamma radiation*
2.5 Mrads sterilizes rubber and most plastics but is not suitable for Teflon, butyrl rubber or polyacetal. Resterilization more than once with gamma radiation results in hardening of plastics.

Methods of disinfection

(a) *Pasteurization*
Pasteurization is useful for anaesthetic equipment which is unsuitable for high temperature heat sterilization. It will kill most viruses, fungi, protozoa and non-sporing bacteria, as well as some spore formers in the growing stage, and tubercle bacilli.

(b) *Chemical disinfectants*
These are usually applied for 30 minutes. The concentration used varies with the purpose but in general increasing the concentration increases the efficacy.

The agents used for anaesthetic equipment include (a) chlorhexidine, mainly effective against gram positive staining bacteria, and (b) formaldehyde and alkaline glutaraldehyde, active against gram negative and gram positive bacteria and moderately active against tubercle bacilli and viruses. Other chemical disinfectants such as hexachlorophene, iodine compounds, phenolics and quaternary ammonium compounds (e.g. cetrimide) are not useful for anaesthetic equipment.

Management of specific items of equipment

(a) *The anaesthetic machine*
This should be wiped down with a chemical disinfectant such as chlor-

hexidine with methylated spirits at least weekly but preferably daily and following use for infected cases. It must be particularly thoroughly cleaned after use for any patient infected by bacteria with multiple antibiotic resistance. Ethylene oxide sterilizers large enough to accommodate an anaesthetic machine have been made but are not widely used.

(b) *Circle absorber*
Circle absorbers should be cleaned at least weekly. Those parts which are easily dismantled should be cleaned with hot water and soap or detergent. Valves must be wiped clean, rinsed and dried, great care being taken to reassemble all parts correctly. The latter are often plastic and should be soaked in a solution such as chlorhexidine 1:1000. Metal canisters and the connecting bar between the two canisters can be autoclaved in a high temperature sterilizer. Perspex canisters are disinfected chemically. Plastic parts are liable to heat deterioration and should be thoroughly cleaned and chemically disinfected.

(c) *Corrugated black rubber tubing*
The corrugated black rubber tubing from the circle absorber to the patient, with the attached Y-piece, should be washed with hot water after each operating list and sterilized in a high temperature sterilizer. There is no need to remove the adaptors at each end. The tubing should be replaced when it loses its resilience. Pasteurization is an acceptable alternative if a suitable pasteurizing water bath or a specially designed washer-pasteurizer is available.

(d) *Single-use plastic tubing*
Both the tubing between the circle absorber and the patient, and the tubing attached to the reservoir bag should be discarded when removed from the machine.

(e) *Reservoir bags*
Most reservoir bags deteriorate with repeated steam sterilization. They are therefore best washed and pasteurized daily in a washer-pasteurizer. In the absence of a suitable machine, daily washing by hand in hot running water followed by rinsing inside and out with chlorine disinfectant (200 ppm available chlorine) for 2 minutes, and hanging to drain is recommended. Solutions of available chlorine include Chlorize (0.16% v/v), Milton (2.0% v/v) or White King (0.5% v/v) and powders include Biochlor (6 g/l), Diversol CX (6 g/l) Multichor (2 g/l) or Saf Sol (8 g/l).

(f) *Other circuits*
Most T-piece circuits can be autoclaved while Bain circuits, which are made with plastic components, can be pasteurized. This should be done at least weekly if they are in frequent use.

(g) *Endotracheal tubes*
At extubation the soiled tubes should be placed directly into a special container for soiled apparatus. They should then be washed with hot water and soap before surface mucus has dried. Scrubbing the outside and passing a sterilized bottle brush through the inside is necessary before rinsing, drying, packaging and sterilizing in a high temperature steam sterilizer. If necessary an endotracheal tube may be left soaking in 1% sodium bicarbonate until proper cleaning can be done. Tubes made of latex do not stand steam sterilization well but they may be pasteurized after cleaning by hand. Some brands of plastic endotracheal tubes can be reused a limited number of times although many are supposed to be for one use only. Autoclaving at lower temperature (121°C) for 15 minutes causes less damage and loss of shape than higher temperature autoclaving. Any type of endotracheal tube should be discarded when it develops a tendency to kink or flatten when bent to an angle of 90°C.

(h) *Endotracheal connectors*
Most plastic tubes are now supplied with plastic connectors which can be discarded with the tube although they can withstand limited low temperature autoclaving. Metal and rubber connections between the endotracheal tube and the corrugated tubing should be washed with hot water and soap after each use and steam sterilized. Permanently connected elbows need not be dismantled. Special rubber connectors should be reserved for the curved metal endotracheal adaptors which vary in size according to the endotracheal tube used. These adaptors should be removed before sterilization to prevent expansion of the rubber connector.

(i) *Pharyngeal airways*
Mucus should be removed by scrubbing the outside in soap and hot water and passing a sterilized bottle brush through the inside, before rinsing, drying and sterilizing by steam under pressure.

(j) *Face masks*
Face masks should be scrubbed with soap and hot water. They may be

steam sterilized if the body of the mask is pierced in half a dozen places with a needle to prevent separation of the layers. The plug for the inflatable rim cushions must be removed to prevent damage to the inflatable rim (Fig. 3.11). If this is not done the mask is useless because an airtight fit between the mask and the face cannot be maintained.

(k) *Laryngoscopes*
The blades are thoroughly scrubbed with soap and water. It is usually necessary to remove the bulb and wash separately.

(l) *Humidifiers*
Some components of these can be autoclaved but wiping over with chlorhexidine and methylated spirit or other appropriate chemical has to suffice for the remainder unless ethylene oxide sterilization is available. Bacterial growth is inhibited in humidifiers which have a water temperature of 50–60°C, although this is lower than the disinfecting temperature required for pasteurization (65+°C). The Bennett cascade is an example of such a humidifier.

(m) *Wright respirometers*
These are normally placed on the expiratory limb of a breathing circuit well away from the patient and they constitute a small hazard only. Surface cleaning after use is sufficient. The only suitable method of sterilization would be an ethylene oxide process.

Infected cases

When 'dirty' cases occur any unnecessary equipment or drugs should be removed from the anaesthetic machine and trolley so that they do not become contaminated. Following anaesthesia the machine and equipment used should be decontaminated and cleaned as outlined above.

Particular care with handling of equipment and cleaning is necessary when the patient is infected by organisms resistant to all commonly used antibiotics. This is becoming an increasing problem in hospitals. A detailed account of the procedure to be used for septic cases is given in Appendix 3.

CHAPTER 4

Physiology in relation to anaesthesia and monitoring

Cardiovascular system. Respiratory system. Blood. Kidney. Body fluids. Acid base balance. Intracranial pressure. Temperature regulation. Malignant hyperpyrexia. Hypothermia. The influence of age.

When a patient is anaesthetized various physiological changes occur. The anaesthetist must understand these and know how the drugs he uses modify normal physiology. The signs which are monitored during anaesthesia help the anaesthetist to recognize changes which occur and to correct gross and undesirable changes before harm comes to the patient.

Some aspects of physiology which are relevant to anaesthesia will be outlined and parameters which can be monitored will be discussed.

Cardiovascular system

The important relationships between blood pressure, cardiac output (volume of blood pumped from the left ventricle per minute is about 5–6 l heart rate and stroke volume (volume pumped each beat — about 70 ml) are summarized in Fig. 4.1.

Cardiac output is dependent on heart rate and stroke volume. Stroke volume is dependent on the amount of blood returning to the heart (venous return) and on the contractility of the ventricular muscle (myocardium). The former is influenced by the blood volume and also the capacitance of the circulation (the amount of blood the circulation will hold). It is reflected by the central venous pressure which is usually measured through a cannula in the right atrium (the lowest pressure point in the circulation) or vena cava. If blood has been lost or the patient is dehydrated or has lost fluid from the circulation, the blood volume will

Blood pressure = Cardiac output x Peripheral resistance

Heart rate   x   Stroke volume

Blood volume   Myocardial
and venous   contractility
return (CVP)

Condition of   Degree of   Sympathetic
myocardium   'stretch'   nervous
               (Starling)   stimulation:
                            adrenaline

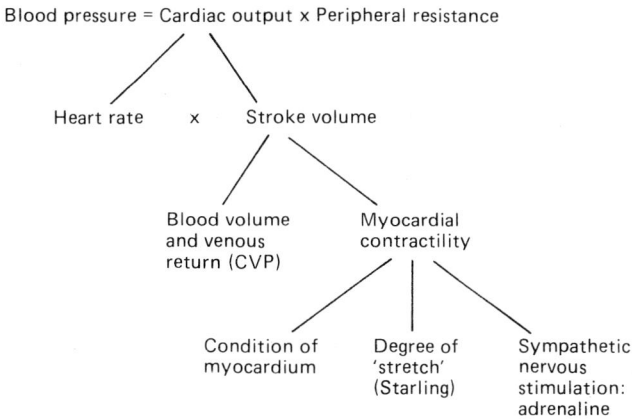

Fig. 4.1   The interplay of cardiovascular factors influencing cardiac output and blood pressure.

be decreased, central venous pressure will be low and stroke volume decreases. In modern discussions this is referred to as reduction in preload. The cardiac output can be maintained initially by increasing heart rate. (The pulse felt on someone who is shocked is rapid and feels thready or soft because stroke volume is reduced.)

The other factor influencing stroke volume is myocardial contractility or how effectively the heart is pumping. The Starling principle is that the more the myocardial fibres are stretched the greater the force of contractions up to a point where disruption of the fibres causes a loss in contractile force. This can be likened to stretching a piece of elastic — the further it is stretched the greater the recoil until it is stretched to breaking point. Thus the more the ventricle fills in diastole (the relaxation phase of the heart) the greater the force of contraction. Conversely, if the blood volume is reduced ventricular filling will be less and the force of contraction will be reduced. If the myocardial fibres are overstretched the heart fails, stroke volume falls and blood is dammed back so that central venous pressure rises.

Myocardial contractility can be depressed by certain drugs (including thiopentone and halothane if too much is given), ischaemia, acidosis or myocardial disease. Ischaemia results from inadequate oxygen supply or obstruction to coronary blood flow. Prolonged ischaemia may result in myocardial infarction. The myocardium is also depressed by an acidosis, which results from the accumulation of an excessive amount of unbuffered hydrogen ion. (See Acid Base Balance below.)

If a drop in stroke volume cannot be compensated by increasing heart rate then cardiac output will fall. Maximum heart rate is lower in old people and the myocardium is less healthy. Their compensating mechanisms will fail sooner and cardiac output is more likely to decline than in younger people. Great care must therefore be taken with drug dosages in the elderly so that overdose is avoided.

If cardiac output declines the sympathetic nervous system which has already caused the tachycardia will increase peripheral resistance. The arterioles become narrower so that the pressure required to push blood through will be greater. The result is that the blood pressure may not fall but the work of the heart is increased so that the myocardium is further strained.

It can be followed from this discussion using Fig. 4.1 that changes in blood pressure may occur quite late when the patient is, for example, bleeding and certainly occur long after the changes in rate and character of the pulse, and a drop in central venous pressure have occurred.

In modern terminology preload refers to ventricular filling where afterload refers to the resistance to blood flow from the heart. Hypertension resulting from chronically increased arteriolar tone and aortic stenosis increase afterload and place an extra strain on the myocardium. Patients with these conditions eventually develop left ventricular failure if not treated. They constitute a group of patients at increased risk during anaesthesia because a drop in cardiac output may result in coronary or cerebral ischaemia.

Anaesthetists frequently have a hand on a pulse during anaesthesia. The value of monitoring rate, pulse pressure and rhythm can be appreciated from the foregoing discussion. Anaesthetists, especially in paediatrics, often use a stethoscope to monitor respiration, and the rate, rhythm and intensity of heart sounds, the latter becoming softer when cardiac output declines. Blood pressure is usually measured and changes commonly occur during anaesthesia. Drugs such as thiopentone, halothane and D-tubocurarine can cause a decrease in blood pressure.

On the other hand some drugs such as ketamine may cause a rise in blood pressure. Sympathetic stimulation resulting in a rise in blood pressure will result from a rise in Pa,co_2 due to hypoventilation, or surgical stimuli if anaesthesia is too light. Thus blood pressure changes can help the anaesthetist know how the patient is responding to the anaesthetic and provide information which will cause the anaesthetist to modify the anaesthetic. A tachycardia and hypertension due to surgical stimulation suggests that the anaesthetic should be deepened or a supplementary analgesic should be given.

Hypotensive anaesthesia can be induced with a vasodilator drug such as intravenous sodium nitroprusside or nitroglycerine. These will relax vascular smooth muscle increasing the volume of blood that can be held in the circulation with a resultant decrease in venous return unless fluids are also given. The hypotension induced by this method will reduce blood loss in operations where blood loss is usually great, thus reducing the amount of blood replacement needed. It may also be useful during surgery on cerebral aneurysms to reduce the likelihood of rupture, and to reduce bleeding so that the surgeon may visualize the operative field better. When this technique is used blood pressure must be monitored carefully so that excessive hypotension which might impair brain and myocardial perfusion does not occur.

An ECG is a record of the electrical activity of the heart which is often monitored, especially in older patients and patients with heart disease. It will show any arrhythmias and evidence of myocardial ischaemia occurring during anaesthesia. When arrhythmias occur the anaesthetist should ascertain the cause and treat them if necessary. If evidence of myocardial ischaemia occurs steps should be taken to improve myocardial oxygenation. These include increasing the inspired oxygen concentration, ensuring ventilation is adequate and treating hypotension or decreased cardiac output.

Respiratory system

During normal respiration the amount breathed in and out with each breath is the tidal volume. This is usually 400–500 ml in an adult and 6–7 ml/kg in infants. The tidal volume can be divided into physiological dead space which is the gas filling the airways that does not take part in gas exchange and the gas which reaches the alveoli that takes part in gas exchange with the blood passing through the lungs — the alveolar ventilation. If the latter is increased, more carbon dioxide is removed and the CO_2 tension in the blood (Pa,co_2) will fall. This decreases the normal stimulus to respiration. The maintenance of a normal Pa,co_2 (40 mmHg) is an important controlling factor in normal respiration. Hypoventilation, with a rise in Pa,co_2 occurs when alveolar ventilation is decreased.

Many anaesthetic drugs and analgesics, such as morphine and pethidine, will cause hypoventilation when larger doses are used if the patient is breathing spontaneously. The presence of hypercarbia (increased Pa,co_2) causes an increase in catecholamine (adrenaline and nor adrenaline) secretion. Some anaesthetics such as halothane and cyclopropane sensitize the myocardium to adrenaline so that arrhythmias may occur when the Pa,co_2 rises. These will usually disappear if ventilation is increased by squeezing the anaesthetic reservoir bag and increasing tidal volume.

When patients are paralysed ventilation is maintained manually by the anaesthetist squeezing the bag or mechanically with a ventilator. Usually the patient is hyperventilated so that Pa,co_2 is lowered. This reduces the tendency to breathe as the action of the muscle relaxant diminishes.

The volume of dead space can be modified by the anaesthetic equipment used. All the gas from where the incoming gas meets the exhaled gas in the circuit constitutes dead space. The use of an ordinary mask increases the dead space significantly. In paediatric anaesthesia special masks (Rendell Baker-Soucek mask) (Fig. 6.7) with a low dead space are used because an increase of, for example, 20 ml will be a much greater relative increase if tidal volume remains the same and dead space increases, alveolar ventilation will decrease and the Pa,co_2 will rise. The opposite can be achieved by intubation of the trachea as the volume of the tube will be less than that of the upper airway.

In some pathological conditions such as emphysema or chronic obstructive airways disease dead space is increased due to destruction of lung tissue so that some gas reaching the lungs does not take part in gas exchange. The important implications of this to anaesthesia are delayed uptake of anaesthetic gases, slowing induction and a chronic inability to get rid of enough CO_2 so that Pa,co_2 is elevated (see Acid Base Balance below). These patients become dependent on low oxygen tension rather than a rising Pa,co_2 to drive respiration. An increase in inspired oxygen may remove their stimulus to respiration and they will stop breathing.

The flow of gases into the lungs depends on the pressure difference between the lungs and the outside atmosphere and also the resistance caused by the size of the airways or endotracheal tube. A narrow tube increases resistance. The volume of gas moved/cm H_2O pressure difference is a measure of compliance. When the lungs are stiff (pulmonary fibrosis) or chest wall is stiff (this occurs in old age) compliance will decrease. When the patient is paralysed with muscle relaxants it becomes easier to inflate the patient by intermittent squeezing of the anaesthetic reservoir bag or with a ventilator because the chest wall compliance is increased. The process of increasing the pressure of gas applied externally so that air enters the lungs is intermittent positive pressure ventilation (IPPV).

The resistance to air flow can be increased by obstruction at any point in the respiratory tract — for example epiglottitis or tumour causing laryngeal obstruction or bronchiolitis or asthma causing lower airways obstruction by narrowing the lumen of the small airways. Increased airways resistance will increase the work of breathing and the respiratory effort. Tracheal tug is a sign of respiratory obstruction. It is a downward movement of the trachea seen in the neck as a depression just above the sternum on inspiration (Fig. 4.2). In infants breathing spontaneously indrawing of the lower rib cage may occur because the costal cartilages are soft and pliable.

Bronchospasm may occur during anaesthesia. This can make it difficult to ventilate the patient even with high inspiratory pressures. Severe bronchospasm can occasionally occur in asthmatics or in patients developing anaphylaxis to a drug given, but lesser degrees are common

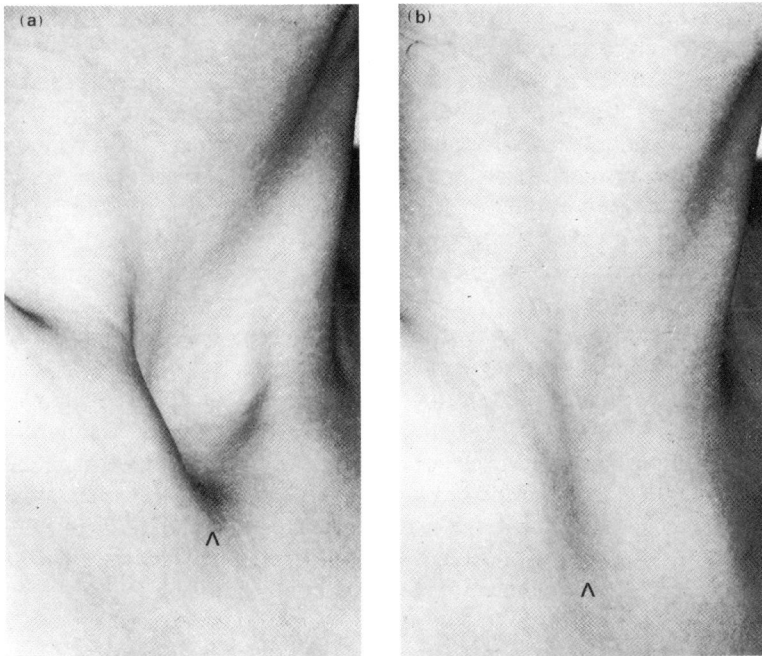

Fig. 4.2 Tracheal tug. The neck immediately above the sternal notch (arrow). (a) During inspiration the negative pressure in the chest sucks the trachea down and the skin over the lower neck inwards if the upper airway is obstructed. (b) With the reduction of negative pressure in the chest during expiration the indrawn tissues return to their resting position.

with drugs such as D-tubocurarine which have a tendency to release histamine in the body.

Anaphylaxis is a severe reaction manifested as bronchospasm and/or hypotension due to capillary damage and leakage of fluid out of the circulation. The patients will have been sensitized by previous exposure to the causative agent.

An anaphylactoid response is similar but the patient has not been previously exposed to the drug. Treatment consists of adrenaline, steroids and intravenous fluids, preferably colloids, if hypotension occurs. Less severe bronchospasm may be relieved by giving the bronchodilator, aminophylline, slowly intravenously. Some anaesthetic agents, particularly ether and methoxyflurane and, to a less extent, halothane have bronchodilating properties which may relieve bronchospasm.

The successful application of intermittent positive pressure ventilation (IPPV) depends on an airtight circuit. Ventilation will not be effective if the patient is paralysed and there is either a large leak or there is a disconnection in the circuit. A disconnection alarm or a pressure gauge in the circuit should detect this. It will not rise if there is a large leak or disconnection in the circuit. If there is an obstruction in the circuit or patient, excessive pressure may be generated. Obstruction to the expiratory side of the circuit can cause dangerous rises in pressure which may result in lung rupture leading to pneumothorax or surgical emphysema.

Ventilation is usually monitored by the anaesthetist watching the chest movement. If the patient is breathing spontaneously the movement of the anaesthetic bag will indicate that the patient is breathing. When the patient is being ventilated by hand much information can be gained by the feel of the bag when compressed. The breath sounds can be monitored with a stethoscope. This is commonly used in children. The volume of ventilation can be measured with a respirometer and the adequacy of ventilation can be checked with a capnograph which measures CO_2 concentration in the expired gas (the end expired CO_2 of 5.6% is equivalent to a normal Pa,co_2 of 40 mmHg), by taking arterial blood or arterialized capillary blood (finger prick) and measuring Pa,co_2.

Blood

Blood is the transport medium for the carriage of oxygen, carbon dioxide, nutrients, waste products of metabolism, hormones and drugs around the body. The effect of a decreased blood volume or cardiac output has already been discussed.

Haemoglobin is important in oxygen transport. One gram of adult haemoglobin (A) carries 1.34 ml of oxygen which is much more than can be carried in simple solution. Thus in anaemia where the haemoglobin is low the capacity for oxygen carriage is reduced. This can only be slightly compensated by increasing the inspired oxygen tension. It is desirable therefore to ensure that patients have a normal haemoglobin before beginning elective surgery. In infancy the haemoglobin is usually high at birth (18-20 g/100 ml) and drops by 3 months to about 11 g/100 ml before gradually rising to the level of 13-14 g/100 ml which is the normal level in adults.

The blood volume increases during the latter half of pregnancy. This is associated with a slight fall in haemoglobin concentration indicating that the plasma volume increases more than red cells and total haemoglobin increase.

When blood loss occurs it is important to maintain blood volume with fluids so that the cardiac output remains normal. Blood transfusion is usually begun when 10-20% of blood volume has been lost but may be begun earlier when continuing large blood loss is expected or if the patient is anaemic preoperatively.

Haemoglobin is usually measured preoperatively so that the anaesthetist can manage the patient appropriately to ensure adequate oxygen carriage.

Kidney

The importance of renal function in anaesthesia is the elimination of drugs and their metabolites and the control function it has on fluid, electrolyte and acid base balance. Hypotension from blood or fluid loss is reflected by diminution of urine flow. Measurement of urine output can be used as one method of assessing the adequacy of fluid replacement because urine production is dependent on an adequate cardiac output and renal blood flow. A urine flow of 0.5-1 ml/kg/hour is indicative of adequate fluid balance.

Body fluids

Water constitutes 60-65% of body weight. About 35-40% is intracellular (about 25 l) and 20-25% is extracellular (about 15 l) of which 4-5% is in plasma. The blood volume is about 70 ml/kg of which 35-40% is red cells (measured as haematocrit). The proportion of water is higher in infants

(75% of body weight) who also have a greater proportion in the extracellular fluid. This and their relatively greater daily fluid turnover makes infants more prone to dehydration than adults.

Electrolyte balance is assessed by measurement of plasma concentrations (Table 4.1) which reflects closely the interstitial fluid concentrations but differs markedly from the intracellular concentrations of electrolytes. In the cells potassium (140–160 mmol/l) and magnesium (30–35 mmol/l) are the main cations (positively charged ions) while phosphate and protein are the main anions (negatively charged ions). If the plasma level of potassium or magnesium is low it may indicate a substantial body deficit. Sodium is the major cation and chloride and bicarbonate are the main anions in the plasma. These are usually measured when electrolyte and acid base measurements are made. In the intracellular fluid the concentration of the latter ions is very low.

Table 4.1   Normal plasma electrolyte levels.

	mmol/l
Sodium	135–143
Potassium	3.7–5.3
Calcium	2.2–2.7
Magnesium	0.7–1.0
Chloride	98–107
Bicarbonate	18–25

When intravenous fluids are ordered the rate of administration should be based on the estimated deficit and maintenance fluid requirements. The latter varies from about 40 ml/kg/day in an adult to about 100 ml/kg/day in a neonate. Electrolyte deficits must be corrected and maintenance amounts should be continued. When the patient's condition and electrolyte results suggest a deficiency in intracellular ions such as potassium or magnesium, additional amounts of these need to be added. They will gradually redistribute into the cells. A deficit of potassium and magnesium is common when the patient is on diuretic therapy and supplements are not given.

Electrolyte imbalance can interfere with the transmission of impulses in nerves, the release of acetyl choline at the neuromuscular junction and in the contraction process in muscle. Electrolyte abnormalities can, therefore, interfere with the response to muscle relaxants and their reversal during anaesthesia.

Acid base balance

The body functions within a very narrow range of free hydrogen ion concentration (H^+). The normal is 40 nmol/l (mol/l $\times$ 10^{-9}). This is a very small amount compared with the concentrations of sodium (0.140 mol/l = 140 mmol/l) or potassium (0.004 mol/l = 4 mmol/l). Unfortunately, the commonly used measure of hydrogen ion concentration is the pH scale which was devised by chemists to simplify the writing of a wide range of concentrations. It is the negative log (H^+) and the normal value is 7.4. Levels below 7.0 (100 nmol/l) and over 8.0 (10 nmol/l) are almost incompatible with survival. (1 mol = 1000 mmol = 1000 000 000 nmol.)

The body is kept close to a pH of 7.4 by buffers, which are substances that can take up free hydrogen ion when there is an excess or release it when there is insufficient without change of pH, so that the amount of free hydrogen ion is kept constant. Examples of these buffer systems are:

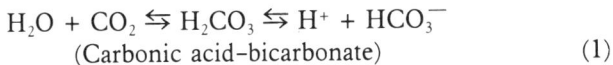

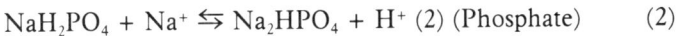

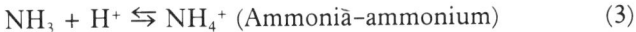

$$H_2O + CO_2 \leftrightarrows H_2CO_3 \leftrightarrows H^+ + HCO_3^-$$
(Carbonic acid–bicarbonate) \hfill (1)

$$NaH_2PO_4 + Na^+ \leftrightarrows Na_2HPO_4 + H^+ \text{ (2) (Phosphate)} \hfill (2)$$

$$NH_3 + H^+ \leftrightarrows NH_4^+ \text{ (Ammonia–ammonium)} \hfill (3)$$

An acidosis occurs when pH falls below 7.4. In blood where pH is usually measured, a pH below 7.4 or a free hydrogen ion concentration above 40 nmol/l is called an acidaemia. An alkalosis is the opposite. A pH above 7.4 or a (H^+) below 40 nmol/l in the blood is an alkalaemia.

Acid base balance is maintained by the lungs and the kidneys. A metabolic or non respiratory problem (e.g. diabetic ketoacidosis or renal failure) leads to accumulation of hydrogen ion and a decrease of bicarbonate. It can only be compensated by the lungs which can remove more carbon dioxide by hyperventilation (a shift to the left in equation 1). It can be seen from Fig. 4.3 that when bicarbonate decreases $P\text{CO}_2$ must decrease if the pH is to remain on the 7.4 pH line.

A patient with emphysema or chronic obstructive airways disease cannot get rid of carbon dioxide normally and develops a high Pa,CO_2. As this rises the patient can only keep on the pH 7.4 line by retaining bicarbonate and excreting more hydrogen ion in the kidney. This is renal compensation for a respiratory problem.

Patients with respiratory failure usually have a Pa,CO_2 above 50 mmHg and if not treated may eventually develop a compensatory metabolic (non-respiratory) alkalosis. Patients with acute respiratory failure

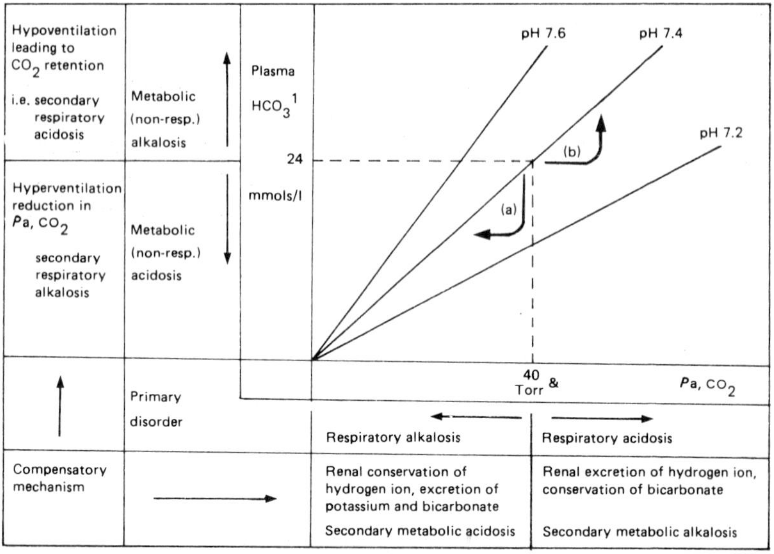

Fig. 4.3 Acid base disturbances and their compensation. (a) The response to metabolic acidosis leading to a reduced Pa,co_2 by hyperventilation (e.g. in diabetic ketoacidosis or renal failure). (b) The increasing plasma bicarbonate in response to CO_2 retention in respiratory disease such as emphysema (chronic obstructive airways disease) or in respiratory failure where Pa,co_2 rises. Torr = mmHg (Pa,co_2).

due to central depression or inadequate respiratory muscle activity are usually treated by artificial ventilation with a respirator set to maintain the Pa,co_2 at or just below 40 mmHg.

When patients are ventilated during anaesthesia it is common to maintain a Pa,co_2 between 30–35 mmHg so that respiratory drive is suppressed. This allows the anaesthetist to control ventilation more easily.

If cardiorespiratory arrest occurs the patient is ventilated to provide oxygen and remove carbon dioxide, and bicarbonate is given to buffer the increasing hydrogen ion accumulating from anaerobic metabolism. Cardiac massage is undertaken to produce some circulation of blood.

Acid base measurements are usually made on arterial blood. pH, Pco_2 and bicarbonate (or base) are usually measured. A base excess indicates a bicarbonate level higher than normal and a base deficit (or negative base excess) indicates a level lower than normal (metabolic or non-respiratory acidaemia).

Intracranial pressure

When the skull is closed intracranial pressure depends on the volumes of the brain, cerebrospinal fluid and blood inside the skull. An increase in the volume of one of these may initially be compensated by decrease in another. As the volume of intracranial contents increase, intracranial pressure rises gradually until the critical volume is reached when pressure rises very rapidly (Fig. 4.4).

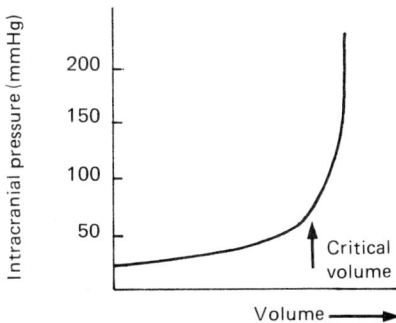

Fig. 4.4 Pressure volume curve showing increasing volume leads to a precipitous rise in intracranial pressure when the critical volume is reached.

The clinical features of raised intracranial pressure include irritability, alteration in conscious state, vomiting, bradycardia, hypertension and respiratory depression. Examination of the eyes by retinoscopy will show the swollen optic discs of papilloedema.

Increasing volume due to tumour, cyst, abscess or cerebral oedema may cause herniation at the tentorium (a dural layer separating the middle from the posterior cranial fossa) or at the foramen magnum (the entrance for the spinal canal into the skull). Tentorial compression causes a progressive decline in the conscious state due to damage to the reticular activating system. This may be accompanied by pupillary and extraocular signs due to compression or stretching of the III, IV and VI cranial nerves.

Herniation at the foramen magnum causes circulatory and respiratory depression due to compression of vital centres in the medulla. Other neurological signs such as weakness or an extensor plantar response are due to compression of nerve tracts running from the brain to the spinal cord.

Intracranial pressure may rise following trauma when brain contusion and cerebral oedema and/or intracranial haemorrhage occur. The frequent observation of the patient's conscious state and neurological signs such as pupillary reflexes is important. Early recognition of rising pressure due to intracranial bleeding may be life saving if burr holes are made promptly to evacuate blood or clot.

Cerebral swelling may also result from infection (encephalitis, meningitis, abscess). Tumours may cause a rise in pressure due to their size or due to obstruction to the normal flow of cerebrospinal fluid leading to cerebral ventricular enlargement. Increased production, obstruction to flow or reduced reabsorption of cerebrospinal fluid may cause raised intracranial pressure except when the sutures are still open in early childhood. In this case separation of the sutures may occur to accommodate the extra volume (hydrocephalus).

Cerebral blood flow is controlled by autoregulation over a wide range of mean arterial pressures (50–160 mmHg). Variation in cerebral vascular tone is controlled primarily by the Pa,co_2 — a high Pa,co_2 causing cerebral vasodilation and an increase in intracranial pressure. On the other hand hyperventilation, by lowering Pa,co_2 and causing vasoconstriction is used by anaesthetists to reduce intracranial pressure during neurosurgery. Hypoxia causes cerebral vasodilation when the Pa,o_2 is below 50 mmHg. Cerebral blood volume may increase in the presence of raised venous pressure or obstructed venous return from the head.

Intracranial pressure becomes atmospheric when the skull is opened but it is important in neurosurgery when the patient has already raised intracranial pressure to prevent further rises. Respiratory depressant drugs such as morphine and pethidine are avoided in the premedication. When the skull is opened the brain may be tense making the operation more difficult. The surgeon can improve the situation by removing cerebro spinal fluid from one of the ventricles. The anaesthetist usually hyperventilates the patient to cause cerebral vasoconstriction. Posture with some head up tilt will aid venous drainage. Avoidance of positive pressure in expiration which also obstructs venous return is also important to prevent increased cerebral blood volume.

If the brain is swollen a diuretic is sometimes used to reduce brain water. Mannitol, an osmotic diuretic, draws water from the brain into the circulation and its osmotic effect also acts in the kidney tubule to reduce reabsorption of water and hence increase urine output. Steroids, particularly dexamethazone, are used to prevent cerebral oedema and are often given before and during surgery for cerebral tumours. They are sometimes used following head injury and may be helpful in minimizing cerebral oedema if given early in large doses.

Anaesthetic drugs influence brain metabolism and cerebral blood flow. Thiopentone reduces cerebral metabolism and hence local carbon dioxide production, provides brain protection during ischaemia, and reduces intracranial pressure. Halothane and other inhalation agents reduce cerebral metabolism but cause cerebral vasodilatation and hence raise intracranial pressure.

Intracranial pressure can be monitored via a ventricular catheter or, more commonly nowadays, by an extradural bolt fixed in a burr hole in the skull. This senses the pressure exerted outwards on the dura by the intracranial contents. These techniques are being used more and more during the intensive care of head injuries and neurosurgical patients.

Temperature regulation

This is normally achieved by skin receptors and others in the hypothalamus in the brain which sense blood temperature. The regulatory mechanisms are depressed by anaesthesia so that heat loss can occur especially during prolonged operations where the abdomen or thorax are open. Infants and small children are particularly prone to cooling because they have little insulation, a small body to act as a heat sink and

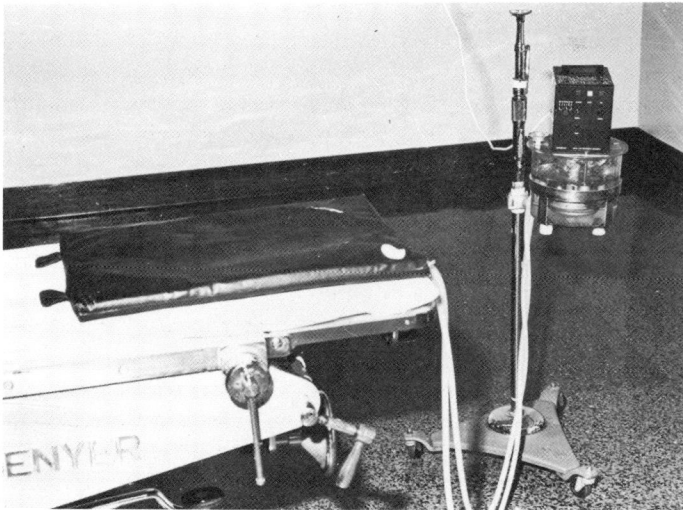

Fig. 4.5 Warm water circulating blanket used to keep patients warm. A more elaborate water temperature controller can be used to cool or warm patients (Heto, Denmark).

a relatively large surface area to body weight ratio compared with adults.

Significant lowering of body temperature delays drug metabolism and recovery from anaesthesia. Several methods of maintaining body temperature during anaesthesia can be used and include warming blankets (usually circulating warm water) under the patient (Fig. 4.5), warming and humidifying the inspired gas by passing it through a humidifier and, especially in neonates, the use of overhead heaters during induction (Fig. 4.6).

The patient's temperature must be monitored when these are in use. When the inspired gases are warmed the temperature should be monitored near the endotracheal tube connector to avoid overheating and burning of the respiratory tract.

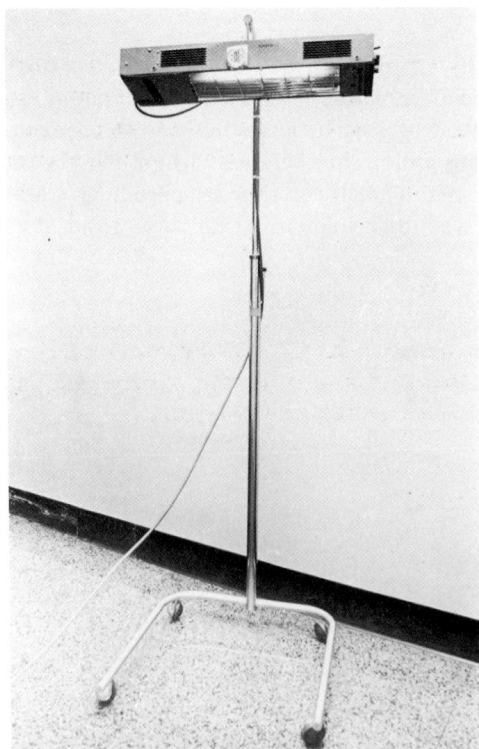

Fig. 4.6 Overhead heater. This mobile heater can be used to keep babies warm during induction of anaesthesia. The height can be adjusted to prevent overheating. A metal measuring tape is attached to the side so that the height above the operating table can be accurately adjusted (75 cm).

Malignant hyperpyrexia

There is a rare hereditary condition called malignant hyperpyrexia where body temperature may rise rapidly to fatal levels on exposure to certain anaesthetics including halothane. Early recognition by temperature monitoring allows time for the institution of life saving measures. These include the administration of oxygen, active cooling with ice packs, gastric lavage with cold water and the administration of cold intravenous solutions, treatment of metabolic acidosis and administration of drugs intravenously. The most effective drug is dantrolene, but procaine has been used with some success in the past.

Hypothermia

Sometimes the body temperature is intentionally lowered — this is called hypothermia. Metabolic rate decreases and allows longer periods of safe circulatory arrest or low blood flow to organs while operating on them (e.g. heart, aneurysms in the cerebral circulation and sometimes in liver surgery — partial hepatectomy).

The influence of age

Patients at the extremes of age — infants and the elderly — vary physiologically and in their response to drugs from the average adult. Some of these differences have already been mentioned.

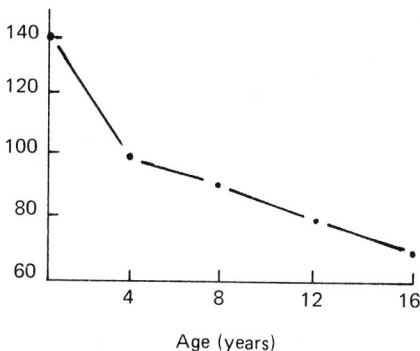

Fig. 4.7 Changes in average rising heart rate with age during childhood.

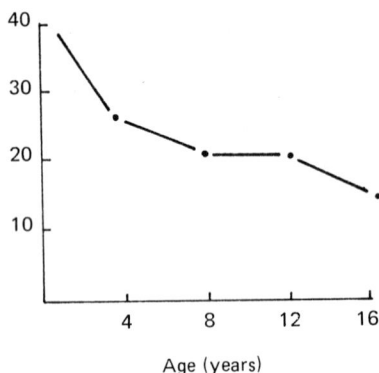

Fig. 4.8 Changes in average resting respiratory rate with age during childhood.

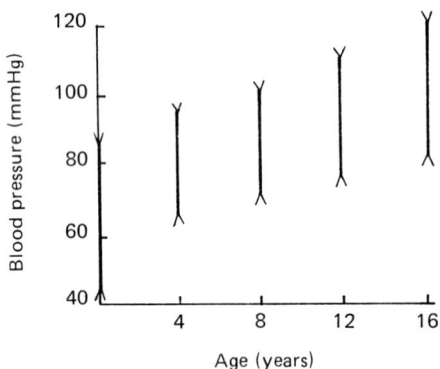

Fig. 4.9 The range of normal blood pressures in children.

Infants have a higher metabolic rate and a greater surface area relative to body weight. As a result cardiac output, heart rate and respiratory rate are greater and gradually decrease with age (Figs. 4.7 and 4.8). Blood pressure tends to be low gradually increasing with age (Fig. 4.9).

At the other end of the age spectrum metabolic rate declines and resting heart rate decreases. Blood pressure gradually rises with advancing age. Compensatory changes in response to physiological stress become less efficient.

The foregoing discussion of physiology provides the rationale for monitoring during anaesthesia. The cardiovascular and respiratory systems are most closely monitored as significant dysfunction may lead to cardiac or respiratory arrest which will lead to death if not promptly treated. A knowledge of the physiology is also important in understanding the relevance of changes which occur in the recovery room and post-operative period.

CHAPTER 5

Drugs used in anaesthesia

History. Use of drugs to produce anaesthesia. Induction agents. Inhalation anaesthetic agents. Muscle relaxants. Atropine and hyoscine. Anticholinesterases. Analgesics. Neuroleptanalgesia. Analgesic antagonists. Local anaesthetics. Antiemetics. Vasodilators. Choice of drugs for anaesthesia. Drug dosage. Complications of drug administration.

History

Humphrey Davy described the potential of nitrous oxide to relieve pain in 1800 but it was not until 1844 that Horace Wells used it for anaesthesia for a dental extraction. A public demonstration by him in 1845 failed because his patient was of the type now known to be very resistant to anaesthetic drugs — a robust, overweight, alcoholic.

Ether was the first agent to be successfully used on a wide scale following a successful demonstration by William Morton at the Massachusetts General Hospital on 16 October 1846. The news travelled fast and the first surgical anaesthetic in Britain was given at Dumfries on 19 December 1846. A dental anaesthetic was given in London on the same day. By June 1847 anaesthetics had been given in Launceston, Tasmania, and Sydney and Newcastle, New South Wales. It is interesting that ether had been used in Georgia, USA, by Crawford Long in 1842, but he did not realize the importance of his discovery and it was not until 1849 that he published his experiences in a medical journal.

In November 1847 chloroform was first used by James Young Simpson to anaesthetize a Gaelic-speaking island boy in Edinburgh.

Among the other interesting stories in the history of anaesthesia are those concerning South American Indian arrow poison described by Sir Walter Raleigh in 1595. From this poison later evolved the muscle relaxant curare. Between 1812 and 1824 Charles Waterton, the Squire of Walton Hall in England, travelled extensively in South America. He injected an arrow poison, wourali, into donkeys. The first one died in 12 minutes. When the second donkey collapsed and stopped breathing, he opened its trachea and kept it alive by ventilating its lungs with a bellows until it recovered — a remarkable forerunner to the introduction of curare and IPPR to anaesthesia in 1942, a century and a quarter later.

Use of drugs to produce anaesthesia

The early anaesthetics were often used as sole agents, rendering the patient both unconscious and pain free. They could also produce muscle relaxation with deeper levels of anaesthesia. Anaesthesia can still be produced in this way but nowadays it is more common to use a combination of drugs which produce good operating conditions with lighter levels of anaesthesia.

Balanced anaesthesia usually consists of a hypnotic to induce anaesthesia (e.g. thiopentone), an analgesic to suppress responses to pain, sometimes an anticholinergic to suppress vagal reflexes (bradycardia and salivation) and a muscle relaxant. The latter keeps the patient still, allows intubation and provides good operating conditions, especially for abdominal surgery, at lighter levels of anaesthesia. Nitrous oxide usually provides some of the analgesia but usually an opiate or another inhalational agent is given as well to ensure that an adequate depth of anaesthesia is achieved so that the patient does not awaken during the operation (Fig. 5.1).

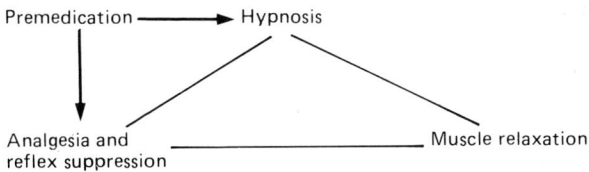

Fig. 5.1   The components of 'balanced' anaesthesia.

Induction agents

These drugs are usually given intravenously and rapidly produce unconsciousness. Their action is brief due either to redistribution of the drug from the brain to other less well perfused tissues thus lowering the brain concentration below the hypnotic level (thiopentone and methohexitone which are ultra short acting barbiturates) or due to the rapid break-down of the drug in the plasma (althesin (Alfathesin) and propanidid (Epontol)). Awakening from the latter two is most rapid, the patients being alert sooner than following thiopentone or methohexitone which are redistributed and then metabolized.

Ketamine can be injected intravenously or intramuscularly. It produces a state of dissociative anaesthesia in which the patient is detached and unaware even though the eyes may remain open. Muscle tone may be increased and movement may occur. It can be used as a sole anaesthetic agent but it can cause unpleasant dreams in some patients, especially if they are disturbed during emergence. This phenomenon occurs more commonly in people who normally dream frequently. Pretreatment with diazepam helps to reduce these undesirable reactions. Its use is now mainly limited to patients with burns and those in regions where full anaesthetic facilities are not available.

Diazepam (Valium) and newer benzodiazapines such as midazolam are sometimes used to induce anaesthesia but the onset of action is slower and less predictable.

Gammahydroxybutyrate (gamma OH) is not widely used but is mentioned because it differs from other agents in that the patients usually take up to 10 minutes to lose consciousness, the drug being metabolized before it becomes active. In young children, where metabolic rate is higher, the onset of anaesthesia is more rapid. It causes prolonged basal anaesthesia.

Inhalation anaesthetic agents

Inhalation anaesthetic agents are gases or vapours which are absorbed from the lungs into the blood and circulated to the tissues, including the brain where their depressant effects make the patient unconscious.

They vary in potency but the concentration required to induce and maintain anaesthesia is known. The anaesthetist uses these concentrations, with modifications depending on the clinical signs observed in the patient, to control the depth of anaesthesia. For instance, if halothane (Fluothane) is being used and the pulse and blood pressure rise on surgical stimulation the concentration may need to be increased. On the other hand halothane causes a dose dependent drop in blood pressure so that if the blood pressure falls excessively the concentration will need to be reduced. Deep halothane anaesthesia also causes respiratory depression.

Nitrous oxide is a weak anaesthetic and needs to be supplemented by an analgesic or other volatile inhalational anaesthetic to provide satisfactory anaesthesia. Inhalation agents vary in their solubility in blood. Those which are relatively insoluble (e.g. nitrous oxide) reach equilibrium between the alveoli, blood and brain quickly while those which are soluble in blood (e.g. methoxyflurane and ether) take a long time to reach equilibrium and it therefore takes longer for the patient to reach the level of anaesthesia necessary for surgery. Halothane and enflurane (Ethrane) are intermediate and can induce anaesthesia fairly rapidly. Using nitrous oxide and oxygen rather than oxygen alone to carry the vapour to the patient hastens induction because nitrous oxide is a weak anaesthetic and it also increases the uptake of the other agent. The latter is called the second gas effect. Using a higher concentration of the inhalation agent initially will also shorten the induction time until surgical anaesthesia is reached. The concentration can then be reduced to maintenance levels.

Some agents are very soluble in fat (halothane and methoxyflurane). In obese patients and when anaesthesia has been prolonged the total amount of anaesthetic in fat will hence be greater than with nitrous oxide. Recovery will be slower due to the amount of drug present and because blood flow to fat is a relatively small part of the cardiac output.

Some agents sensitize the heart to adrenaline and increase the tendency to cardiac arrhythmias if the surgeon uses it as a vasoconstrictor. This occurs with halothane which should be avoided when adrenaline is to be injected.

Ether and cyclopropane are flammable and are rarely used now because of the widespread use of diathermy. Both were very popular and useful agents in the past and ether is still commonly used in underdeveloped countries as it is cheap and easily transportable, provides good operating conditions and is relatively safe as it is not easy to overdose the patient.

Inhalation agents vary in the degree of hypnosis, analgesia, reflex depression and muscle relaxation they produce although all can usually be achieved with deep levels of anaesthesia. The problem is that the deeper the anaesthetic the more prolonged the postoperative period of unconsciousness, the greater the incidence of postoperative vomiting and the greater the risk of cardiac or respiratory arrest. Table 5.1 summarizes the actions of commonly used agents. When comparing potency, anaesthetists use the concentration needed to abolish response to surgical stimuli in 50% of subjects. This is called the minimum alveolar

Table 5.1 Summary of the properties of inhalational anaesthetic agents.

Drug	BP°C	Solubility in blood	Rate of induction	Solubility in fat	Rate of emergence	Maintenance concentration	Hypnotic	Analgesia	Muscle relaxation	MAC %	Compatibility with adrenaline	Other properties
Halothane (Fluothane)	50.2	Moderate (2.3)	Fairly rapid	High	Fairly rapid but delayed after prolonged anaesthesia	0.5–2%	++	+	++	0.74	No	May cause laryngeal spasm especially in children. BP lowers with higher doses
Nitrous oxide	(–88) gas at room temp.	Insoluble (0.47)	Rapid	Low	Rapid	Usually about 70% used as supplement to other agent or narcotic	+	+++	—	105	Yes	Must be supplemented to produce anaesthesia
Enflurane (Ethrane)	57	Moderate (1.9)	Fairly rapid	Moderate	Fairly rapid	1.5–4%	++	++	++	1.7	No	Depress and with IPRR. Laryngeal spasm occasionally in children
Methoxyflurane (Penthrane)	104	Very soluble (13)	Slow	High	Slow	0.25–1%	++	++++	+++	0.16	No	Bronchodilator. Potent smell. Nephrotoxic with prolonged use
Trichlorethylene (Trilene)	87	Soluble (9)	Slow	High	Slow	0.1–0.3%	++	++++	+	0.17	No	Contains blue colouring. Should not be used with soda lime
Ether	35.5	Very soluble (12)	Slow	Moderate	Slow	3–12%	++	++++	+++	1.9	Yes	Flammable Bronchodilator

concentration (MAC). In practice the concentration used to anaesthetize patients will be greater than MAC unless other agents such as nitrous oxide or analgesics are used at the same time to ensure that the patient is adequately anaesthetized.

Muscle relaxants

These drugs act by blocking transmission at the neuromuscular junction so that a nerve stimulus does not cause a muscle contraction. The muscles, including those used in breathing, thus become paralysed. It is therefore essential to inflate the lungs rhythmically by positive pressure ventilation until the paralysis has worn off. Normally a nerve impulse releases acetyl choline from the nerve ending and this attaches to the receptor site on the muscle where it initiates cell depolarization and muscle contraction.

There are two types of neuromuscular blocking drugs — depolarizing and non depolarizing (Fig. 5.2). Suxamethonium (Scoline and Anectine) is a depolarizing relaxant which has a chemical structure

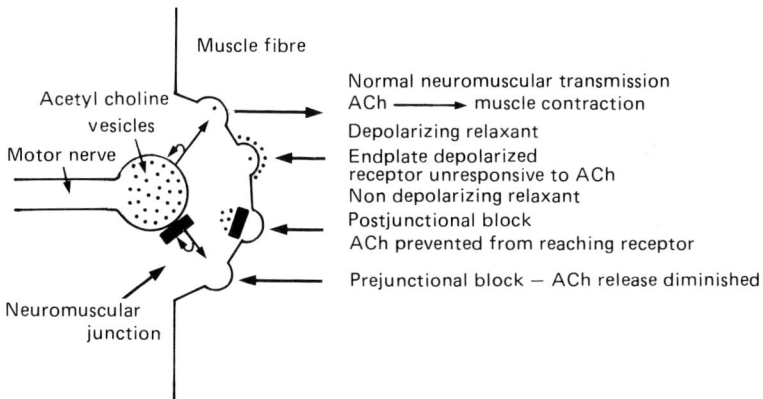

Fig. 5.2 Diagrammatic representation of the neuromuscular junction. Normal transmission — acetyl choline (ACh) released from granules in nerve ending. Some attaches to receptor causing neuromuscular transmission of impulses. Some acts back on nerve ending to promote further release of ACh (+ve feedback). Suxamethonium attaches to receptor causing depolarization. Non-depolarizing relaxants prevent access of ACh to receptor. D-tubocurarine is now thought also to interfere with the +ve feedback loop thus decreasing ACh release.

resembling two acetylcholine molecules stuck together. It mimics the effect of acetylcholine causing depolarization at the receptor but instead of causing a very transient effect on the receptor as acetylcholine does, before it is broken down by cholinesterase, suxamethonium alters the sensitivity of the receptor site so that it does not respond to acetyl choline for 3–5 minutes during which time the muscle remains paralysed. Suxamethonium is broken down by pseudocholinesterase when it leaves the receptor site.

Muscle fasciculations are commonly seen during depolarization, especially in adults. Muscle pains are a common complication following suxamethonium especially if the patient does not rest postoperatively. This is probably due to muscle fibre damage during depolarization as opposing muscles do not relax and contract synchronously but depolarize and contract randomly. A small number of the population have genetically inherited variants of pseudocholinesterase which do not break down suxamethonium normally. The result is prolonged paralysis and the patient's lungs will have to be ventilated until the paralysis wears off.

Suxamethonium in normal doses can cause cardiac arrest due to excessive potassium release during depolarization in severe burns and following severe trauma. The hazard is greatest for a varying period

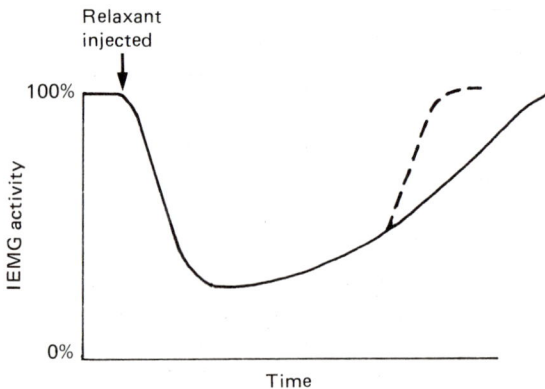

Fig. 5.3 An integrated electromyogram (IEMG) showing the reduction in activity following the administration of neuromuscular blocker. The degree of depression is related to the number of receptors occupied by the muscle relaxant. Recovery occurs as the drug gradually leaves more and more receptors. This process can be hastened (dotted line) by the administration of an anticholinesterase such as neostigmine. (Usually given with atropine which prevents undesirable parasympathetic effects.)

between 1 and 6 weeks following injury. It can be avoided by markedly reducing the dose of suxamethonium (e.g. to 0.2 mg/kg).

Non-depolarizing relaxants, D-tubocurarine (Tubarine), alcuronium (Alloferin), gallamine (Flaxedil) and pancuronium (Pavulon), prevent acetyl choline reaching the receptor rather than mimicking its action. There is thus no contraction before relaxation. The period of paralysis is longer, about 15–30 minutes, depending on the dose and is longest with D-tubocurarine. Gradually the relaxant leaves the receptor site and more and more receptors recover their activity. This can be demonstrated with an integrated EMG recording where the height of the muscle action potentials in response to stimulation of the nerve is inversely related to the number of receptors occupied (Fig. 5.3).

The action of non-depolarizing relaxants can be reversed by giving an anticholinesterase. This blocks cholinesterase so that the breakdown of acetylcholine is slower. The increasing concentration of acetylcholine overcomes the effect of non-depolarizing (competitive) muscle relaxant with rapid return of muscle power. The anticholinesterase commonly used is neostigmine. This also causes an increase in acetylcholine at

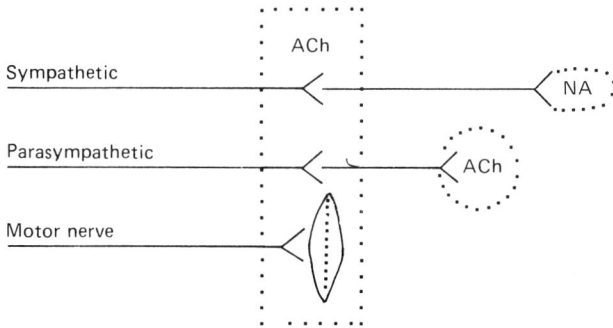

Fig. 5.4 Sites of action of acetylcholine (ACh). Ganglia, neuromuscular junction (nicotinic) and parasympathetic postganglionic nerve endings (muscarinic). Noradrenaline (NA) is the transmitter at sympathetic postganglionic nerve endings. Acetylcholine also acts in the central nervous system. Atropine blocks the action of acetylcholine at parasympathetic endings.

autonomic ganglia and parasympathetic postganglionic nerve endings (Fig. 5.4). The resulting parasympathetic stimulation causes bradycardia, salivation and gut contraction which are undesirable and hazardous, so that atropine is always given before or with the neostigmine to block these parasympathetic effects.

Atropine and hyoscine

Atropine and hyoscine are the two most commonly used anticholinergic drugs. Atropine has more potent peripheral effects, blocking the para-sympathetic receptors on the end organ. It thus increases heart rate, reduces secretions from glands, diminishes gut contractility and dilates the pupil. Hyoscine (scopolamine) exhibits these actions to a lesser degree but it is a more powerful antisialogogue (antisalivation) and has more effect on the central nervous system causing sedation and amnesia. It is thus commonly used in premedication.

Anticholinesterases

Anticholinesterases block the enzyme cholinesterase and enhance the effects of acetylcholine. Neostigmine (Prostigmine) acts predominantly at peripheral sites (autonomic ganglia, parasympathetic nerve endings and the neuromuscular junction) and is used commonly to reverse neuromuscular blocking drugs. Physostigmine (Eserine) can cross the blood brain barrier and has greater central effects. Its uses include reversing postoperative delirium and confusion, hastening arousal following gammahydroxybutyrate and, in intensive care, stopping convulsions and lightening coma following tricyclic antidepressant and anti-histamine overdosage.

Analgesics

Morphine and papaveretum (Omnopon) are the oldest potent analgesics in common use. Their advantages are that they also provide some psychic sedation and euphoria and they are cheap. Their disadvantages, shared with others in this group, are that they can cause addiction, respiratory depression and increased nausea and vomiting in surgical patients. Pethidine is a synthetic analgesic with similar properties but it causes less psychic sedation and euphoria than morphine.

Pentazocine (Fortral) is a non-addicting, strong analgesic but is also an analgesic antagonist. It should not be used before the other analgesics because it will reduce their effect.

Neuroleptanalgesia

Phenoperidine and fentanyl are analgesic drugs with a shorter duration of action (except when used in very large doses) and are used with droperidol to produce neuroleptanalgesia. They are also used as intra-operative analgesic supplements largely because of their shorter duration of action. Fentanyl has less effect on blood pressure than pethidine and phenoperidine.

Droperidol (Droleptan) is a tranquilizer with antiemetic properties, and it produces a detached state of mind which can be disturbing to the patient unless another drug is used with it. Neuroleptanalgesia is used for some investigations, such as neuroradiological procedures in adults, allowing the patient to be comfortable and sedated but still cooperative and responsive to commands. The addition of nitrous oxide provides light general anaesthesia.

Analgesic antagonists

Several drugs structurally similar to morphine can antagonize or reverse the action of the strong analgesics. The most effective and widely used is naloxone (Narcan). Patients with central depression or hypoventilation who have had analgesics pre- or intraoperatively are usually rapidly aroused by naloxone. Care must be taken not to give too much because complete reversal of the analgesic effect will result in the patient feeling pain.

Local anaesthetics

These drugs act on nerves to block the transmission of nerve impulses. Sensory and motor nerves may both be blocked although the degree of block of these varies with different drugs. Of the two long acting drugs, bupivacaine (Marcaine) produces a predominantly sensory block with motor block when a higher concentration (0.5%) is used while etidocaine tends to produce more motor block (i.e. the muscles are relaxed more). These drugs last 4–12 hours depending on the site of injection and have led to increasing use of local anaesthetic blocks (such as epidural, caudal or intercostal blocks) for postoperative analgesia.

The most widely used local anaesthetic is lignocaine (Xylocaine) which lasts from 1 to 2 hours. Other local anaesthetics include prilocaine (Citanest), which can cause methaemoglobinaemia and make patients look cyanosed when doses exceeding 8–9 mg/kg are given, mepivacaine (Carbocaine), procaine, which is short acting and is the oldest one still in use, and cinchocaine (Nupercaine) which is used mainly for spinal anaesthesia.

Adrenaline is sometimes added to local anaesthetics to cause vasoconstriction of the blood vessels in the area where they are injected. The resulting reduced blood flow slows the uptake of local anaesthetic from the site. This results in a longer action and reduces the likelihood of toxic blood levels being reached. It is dangerous to use adrenaline with local anaesthetics for digital or penile blocks. The arteries in the area are end arteries and if they become constricted ischaemia may result with tissue loss.

The major toxic effects of local anaesthetics are convulsions and bradycardia. They are most likely to occur with excessive doses or following accidental intravenous injection. When convulsions occur the patient should be ventilated with oxygen, and only when they persist should an anticonvulsant be given. Thiopentone is often used for this purpose as it is usually readily available when local anaesthetic toxicity occurs. Diazepam effectively suppresses convulsions produced by local anaesthetics.

Antiemetics

These are drugs which reduce nausea and vomiting. Following anaesthesia 10–50% of patients vomit. The incidence is higher following some operations such as those involving the middle ear. In others, such as open eye operations vomiting will raise intraocular pressure and as this is undesirable attempts should be made to prevent it.

Most antiemetics act on the vomiting centre in the brain stem (medulla) which includes the chemoreceptor trigger zone. These include many of the phenothiazines such as chlorpromazine (Largactil), promethazine (Phenergan), prochlorperazine (Stemetil) and trifluperazine (Trilafon). The phenothiazines, especially chlorpromazine, promethazine and trimeprazine, also have sedative and tranquilizing effects which are useful in premedication and some antihistamine activity. Hyoscine and droperidol which are commonly used in anaesthesia also have antiemetic properties.

Metoclopramide (Maxolon) stimulates gastric emptying and has a central action on the vomiting centre. As well as its use as a postoperative antiemetic it is sometimes used prior to emergency surgery to hasten stomach emptying and reduce the chances of vomiting and aspiration during induction.

Vasodilators

Vasodilators are sometimes used during anaesthesia to lower blood pressure and thus reduce bleeding. This is called induced hypotension. The drugs which produce this effect either act directly on the vascular smooth muscle (e.g. sodium nitroprusside and nitroglycerine), block transmission at sympathetic ganglia (trimetaphan) or block the sympathetic vasoconstrictor receptors (e.g. phentolamine and phenoxybenzamine). The former are more commonly used in anaesthesia by intravenous infusion because they are short acting and the blood pressure will rise rapidly after they are discontinued.

Choice of drugs for anaesthesia

There are usually several ways to achieve anaesthesia for a particular operation. The drugs selected for a particular anaesthetic will depend on the duration and nature of the operation, the anaesthetist's preference based on his experience with the drugs and their relevant properties and to some degree on the patient's condition and preference. For instance, it is inappropriate to use an induction agent in a dose which will significantly lower blood pressure in a patient with aortic stenosis because it will result in reduced coronary blood flow and possibly myocardial ischaemia or infarction.

Some patients may express a preference, for example, for a regional rather than a general anaesthetic and many children prefer to breathe a gas to go to sleep than to have a needle for an intravenous induction.

Drug dosage

Commonly used doses of many of the drugs discussed are summarized in Table 5.2. Doses are often quoted for average adults despite the fact that adults vary widely in size and weight. Thus the average total dose should be reduced in small thin people, in the elderly, cachectic or very ill; generally increased in large people, although if the excess weight is fat the increase should be less than in a large lean person; and modified

Table 5.2 Commonly used doses of drugs used in anaesthesia.

Group	Drug	Dose/kg		Comment
Induction agents	Thiopentone	4–5	mg i.v.	Less needed in shock and elderly, more if apprehensive
	Methohexitone	2	mg i.v.	
	Alfathesin	0.05–0.07	ml i.v.	
	Propanidid	5–7	mg i.v.	
	Ketamine	(1–4	mg i.v.	Dose related to duration of action required
		(4–10	mg i.m.	
	Gamma OH	30–70	mg i.v.	Sleep 1–2 hours
Muscle relaxants	d-tubocurarine	0.6–0.7	mg i.v.	Dose reduced in neonates and in obese because patients
	Alcuronium	0.3	mg i.v.	have smaller proportion of muscle
	Gallamine	3.0	mg i.v.	
	Pancuronium	0.08	mg i.v.	
	Suxamethonium	1.0	mg	Causes muscle twitches
Anti-cholinergics	Atropine	0.01–0.025	mg	Dose usually half neostigmine
				dose when used in combination
	Hyoscine	0.008	mg	
Anti-cholinesterases	Neostigmine	0.03–0.05	mg i.v.	
	Physostigmine	0.03–0.05	mg i.v.	
Analgesics	Morphine	0.2	mg i.m.	
	Papaveretum	0.3–0.4	mg i.m.	
	Pethidine	1.0	mg i.m.	
	Pentazocine	0.5	mg i.m.	

Category	Drug	Dose	Unit	Notes
	Phenoperidine	0.01–0.02	mg i.v.	Duration of action related to dose. High doses sometimes used during anaesthesia
	Fentanyl	1–3	μg i.v.	
Neurolept	Droperidol	0.015	mg i.v.	
Analgesic antagonist	Naloxone			Dose used is one which produces desired effect
Local anaesthetic (maximum dose without adrenaline)	Lignocaine	5	mg	The doses are for injection (not i.v.). Higher maximum doses can be used when adrenaline is used to slow absorption
	Procaine	10–14	mg	
	Mepivicaine	5	mg	
	Prilocaine	5	mg	
	Bupivacaine	2	mg	
	Etidocaine	4	mg	
Antiemetics	Chlorpromazine (Largactil)	0.5	mg i.m.	
	Promethazine (Phenergan)	0.5	mg i.m.	
	Prochlorperazine (Stemetil)	0.1	mg i.m.	
	Metoclopramide (Maxalon)	0.15–0.2	mg i.m.	Total daily dose not to exceed 0.5 mg/kg

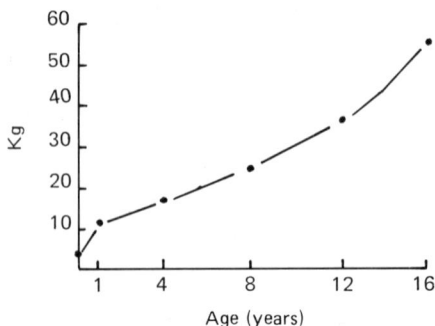

Fig. 5.5 The average increase in body weight with age in children. A useful formula which can be used as a guide is 2 × age + 9 kg from 1 to 8 years and 3 × age kg from 8 to 13 years.

according to age and weight in a child (Fig. 5.5). It would be logical to work on an approximate dose/kg but this is done much less commonly for adult patients than children. Neonates are sensitive to many drugs and require much smaller doses.

Complications of drug administration
(a) *Overdosage*
This can occur following an excessive dose or as a result of more rapid absorption resulting in high blood levels being reached. In anaesthesia the most serious are cardiovascular and respiratory depression which can occur following overdose with most intravenous, inhalation and local anaesthetic agents. Another complication of overdosage is prolongation of the action of the drug with delayed recovery from anaesthesia.

(b) *Site of injection*
Sometimes drugs are inadvertently injected into the wrong site. Intra-arterial injection of thiopentone can cause vasospasm of surrounding tissues. When this happens the needle should be left in the artery, the drug diluted by flushing with saline and then a small dose of the anti-coagulant heparin is injected to prevent thrombosis. Spasm can be relieved with a vasodilator such as sodium nitroprusside (0.02 mg/kg) or papaverine (0.5 mg/kg in 20 ml saline) and procaine (0.2 mg/kg), 0.5% solution can be injected to relieve pain. Sometimes a stellate ganglion block is performed to block the sympathetic vasconstrictor nerves to the arm.

Neuritis can follow the traumatic injection of local anaesthetic or inadvertent injection of other drugs such as thiopentone into a nerve. This can occasionally be debilitating and painful for several months. Accidental intravenous injection of local anaesthetics may lead to acute toxicity. Total spinal anaesthesia resulting in loss of consciousness, respiratory paralysis and hypotension can result from inadvertent injection of local anaesthesia into the subarachnoid instead of the epidural space. The volume used epidurally is much greater than that needed for spinal anaesthesia.

The volume of local anaesthetic required for epidural analgesia in late pregnancy is less than in a non-pregnant patient. The reason for this is thought to be the distension of the epidural veins during pregnancy.

Some drugs are irritant when injected accidentally subcutaneously. Thiopentone, especially a 5% solution which is rarely used now, may cause sloughing of the overlying skin.

(c) *Pharmacogenetic variants*
Some patients exhibit an undue sensitivity to a drug. This may be due to an inherited condition in which the patient has an enzymatic defect or variant from normal. Examples include the following:

1 The abnormal cholinesterases which do not break down suxamethonium normally resulting in prolonged paralysis.

2 Acute intermittent porphyria — barbiturates can cause an exacerbation leading to neurological complications, paralysis and respiratory failure.

3 Malignant hyperpyrexia — on exposure to a variety of anaesthetic drugs there is excessive muscle activity and the body temperature rises rapidly, often with fatal results unless treated promptly. (See Chapter 4 Temperature Regulation)

(d) *Allergy and anaphylaxis*
Atopic individuals may develop complications such as bronchospasm more readily, especially following drugs which release histamine. Some people become sensitized to a drug and may develop a rash, urticaria, or in the most severe cases anaphylaxis where bronchospasm and/or severe hypotension can result from leakage of fluid from capillaries into the tissues. Treatment includes adrenaline 1:10 000 intravenously and colloid fluids intravenously for hypotension. Anaphylactoid reactions are similar but occur without previous exposure. These reactions may be life threatening and, although rare, can occur with many drugs used in anaesthesia.

(e) *Patient disease*

Apart from genetic diseases patients with certain diseases exhibit altered sensitivity to some drugs. Hypothyroid patients may be very sensitive to depressant drugs and develop hypotension and have delayed recovery from anaesthesia. Patients on high dose steroids or with Cushings syndrome may have a reduced stress response and become hypotensive with anaesthesia.

(f) *Phlebitis*

Some drugs injected intravenously cause phlebitis and sometimes thrombosis near the site of injection. It does not usually become apparent for several days. The incidence can be reduced by dilution of the drugs.

(g) *Nephrotoxicity*

This occurs following prolonged anaesthetics with methoxyflurane (usually exceeding 2 hours at concentrations above MAC or 0.16%). It will develop with lower total dose if the patient is on another nephrotoxic drug such as gentamicin. It is due to the release of inorganic fluoride during methoxyflurane metabolism. It is unlikely to occur in children.

(h) *Hepatotoxicity*

Some halogenated hydrocarbon inhalation anaesthetics have been suspected of causing liver damage. Chloroform sometimes caused centrilobular necrosis. Much debate has occurred about the possible hepatotoxic effect of halothane. It may cause some damage if the patient is malnourished, hypoxia occurs or on repeated exposure in sensitive individuals. Often other causative factors may be present in patients who develop postoperative jaundice.

In summary, the nature and use of drugs commonly used in anaesthesia has been outlined in this chapter. Some basic general principles have been discussed so that the reason for the way the drugs are used can be appreciated and important complications have been outlined. For a full description of the drugs further details can be obtained from more comprehensive text books of anaesthesia and pharmacology.

CHAPTER 6

The conduct of anaesthesia including the role of the anaesthetist's assistant

The assistant. Checking the equipment. Intravenous infusions. Drugs. Monitoring equipment. Induction and the establishment of anaesthesia. Intubation. Application of cricoid pressure. Posturing the patient. The positioning of the anaesthetist. Application of diathermy and electrical equipment. Maintenance of general anaesthesia. Regional anaesthesia. Conclusion of general anaesthesia. Chest drains. Transfer to recovery room.

The assistant

Assistance is usually provided by an anaesthetic technician, nurses who are specially trained or nursing staff working in the operating theatre. It is important that the anaesthetist has an assistant, preferably with experience, when beginning and concluding an anaesthetic. There are also times during the procedure when the anaesthetist needs an extra person to help.

The role of the assistant includes preparing the equipment and machine, setting up intravenous equipment if necessary and handing equipment such as the laryngoscope and endotracheal tube to the anaesthetist when the patient is going to be intubated. He or she may help attach monitoring devices and the diathermy plate and may be involved with positioning the patient on the operating table.

Checking the equipment

Before an anaesthetic or operating list is started the equipment should be checked and the items needed should be laid out clean and ready for use. Defective equipment may lead to inability to ventilate the patient. Errors in flowmeter connection of gas lines and supplies can lead to hypoxic gas mixtures being supplied. Safety checks and modern connections are aimed to prevent these problems.

The gas supply and cylinders should be checked to ensure that oxygen and nitrous oxide are available and that the oxygen supply warning device (e.g. Bosun) is working. The machine should be checked to ensure that the rotameter bobbins are rotating, that the vapourizers contain a sufficient amount of the correct liquid anaesthetic and that it can be turned on and off. The circuit should be checked for leaks by turning on the oxygen, and occluding the common gas outlet. The rotameter bobbin should fall if there are no leaks. The appropriate circuit should be chosen and it should be ensured that the gas supply is connected. If a circle system is to be used check that the soda lime is not exhausted, that the breathing hoses and bags are correctly assembled and that the valves function. Although checking the gas supply, especially cylinders, the level of anaesthetic in the vapourizer and the soda lime is often undertaken by the assistant it is the legal responsibility of the anaesthetist to ensure the equipment is functioning properly before beginning an anaesthetic.

The assistant usually ensures that the masks and laryngoscopes are clean and that the latter are in working order (there should always be two on hand) and that the appropriate sterile endotracheal tubes are available and ready for use.

Intravenous infusions

If an intravenous infusion is required this must be set up. The basic intravenous set may have additional items added. If rapid transfusion is

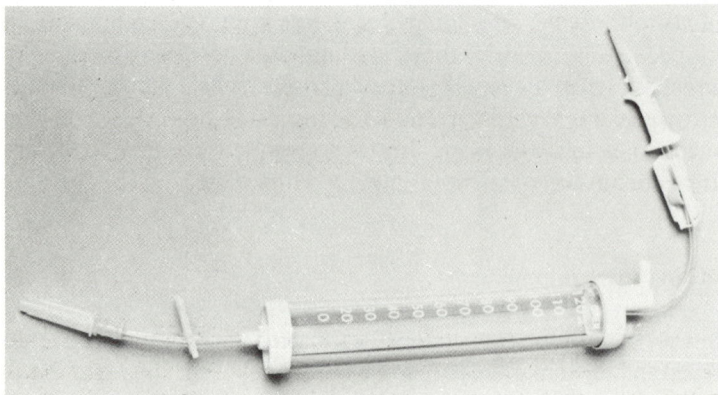

Fig. 6.1   A burette for measuring small volumes of fluids during intravenous infusions in children.

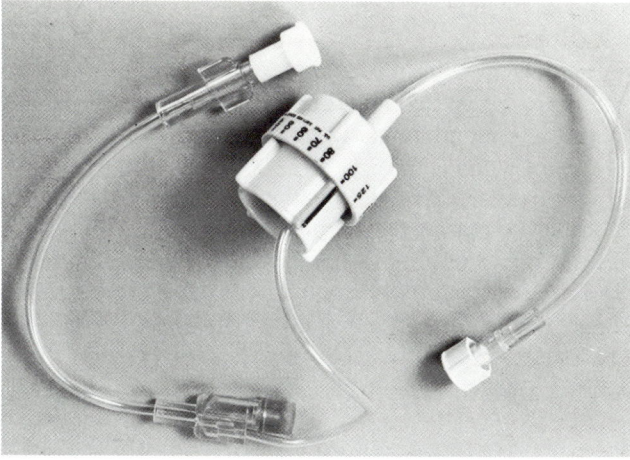

Fig. 6.2   A 'dial-a-flow' device for fine control of intravenous infusions. It is cheaper than the more sophisticated syringe and roller pumps.

likely to be required a pump set in the line can be used to increase the infusion rate and a coil and blood warmer can be inserted so that if large volumes of blood or fluid are given they can be warmed. Cold blood given rapidly can cause cardiac arrest. A burette to measure small volumes (mainly in children under 15–20 kg) (Fig. 6.1), a three way tap, an extension set and possibly a flow rate control such as Dial-a-flow or a pump (Fig. 6.2) when a drug infusion is to be used may also be added. All these add to the cost and should only be used if really necessary. The fluid to be used will be decided by the anaesthetist and should be checked by him (see Chapter 7). An accurate record of fluid and blood given and blood loss and urine output should be kept so that fluid balance can be easily assessed.

Drugs

When drugs are drawn up the syringe should be labelled and the concentration indicated if the drug is diluted. The anaesthetist is legally responsible for all drugs administered. The syringes and needles should be kept on a sterilized tray separate from the laryngoscope and other dirty equipment.

Monitoring equipment

The appropriate monitoring equipment should be made ready. For more complex surgery additional items such as transducers for intravascular pressure monitoring will need to be sterilized and the equipment calibrated.

When the patient is brought into the anaesthetic room (or operating theatre) a blood pressure cuff is placed on the arm. In children the correct size covers two-thirds of the upper arm. Wider ones will record a lower pressure and narrower ones a higher pressure than the real value. Other items such as ECG leads and a stethoscope can be attached. A precordial stethoscope should be strapped on to the chest firmly (Fig. 6.3) to ensure good contact.

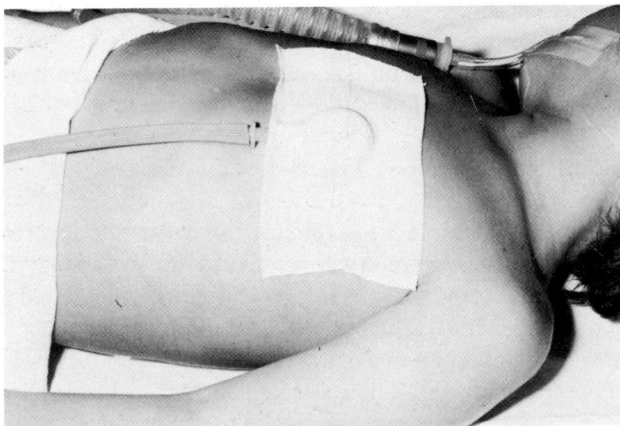

Fig. 6.3 The stethoscope head attached to the precordium with elastoplast. This method usually maintains good contact so that variations in heart sounds due to varying contact between the stethoscope and skin are minimized.

Induction and establishment of anaesthesia

While the patient is conscious in the induction room idle chatter amongst staff should be avoided. Staff in attendance should show concern for the patient and be sensitive to his or her anxiety. As anaesthesia is about to commence it is better for the anaesthetist to conduct any conversation with the patient that may be necessary.

Anaesthesia can be induced by (a) an intravenous injection, e.g. thiopentone, althesin, etc, (b) inhalation of anaesthetic gases, e.g. nitrous oxide and halothane, (c) occasionally intramuscularly, e.g. ketamine, and (c) rarely by rectal administration of thiopentone or methohexitone. Formerly the whole anaesthetic was given with an inhalational agent using a mask, but modern anaesthesia usually employs a number of drugs so that lighter levels of anaesthesia can be maintained while still providing good operating conditions. Figure 5.1 summarizes the main components — hypnosis, analgesia and reflex suppression and muscle relaxation. The premedication can provide a part of the anaesthetic by reducing the requirements of hypnotic and analgesic.

(a) *Intravenous induction*
This is usually a pleasant, rapid method of induction. The availability of fine sharp needles reduces the discomfort from the venepuncture. Once an intravenous needle or cannula is in place relaxants and other other drugs can easily be given. The winged needles with extension tubing, such as the 'butterfly', can be left *in situ* for injections without an intravenous infusion attached if one is not needed (Fig. 6.4).

Prior to venepuncture the assistant can apply a tourniquet or use a hand to act as a tourniquet. The aim is to occlude venous but not arterial flow so that the veins distend. Tapping over the vein or flexing the wrist a few times increases the venous distension (Fig. 6.5). Angled light makes

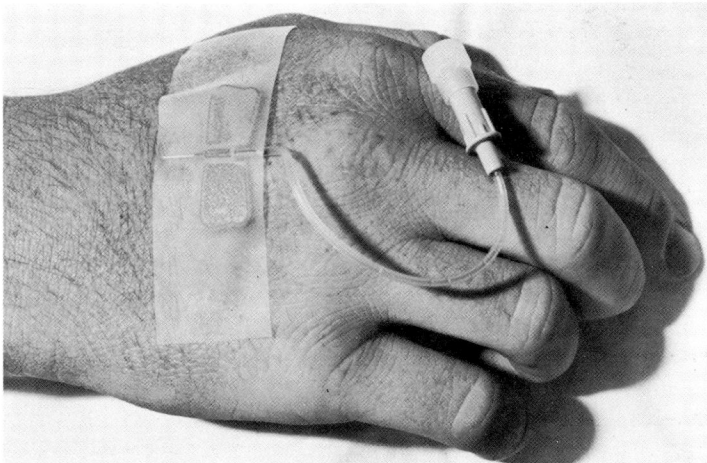

Fig. 6.4 A 'butterfly' needle can be plugged off and kept in a vein allowing easy intravenous access for drug administration.

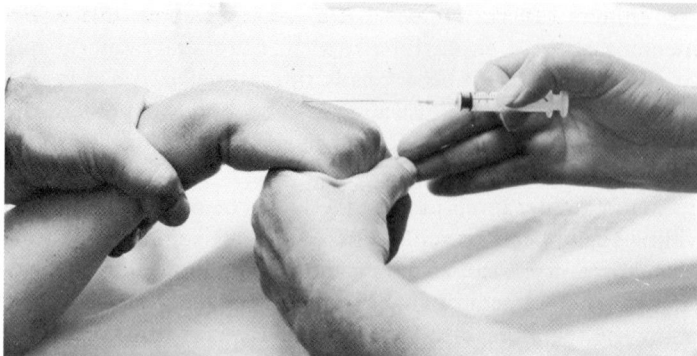

Fig. 6.5   Insertion of an intravenous cannula. An assistant can constrict the wrist putting proximal traction on the skin while the anaesthetist flexes the wrist so that the vein is taut but not collapsed. Angled lighting throws a shadow which makes it easier to see the vein as is demonstrated here. Alternatively a tourniquet can be used.

the distended vein more obvious. When the hand is used as a tourniquet in children ensure that the patient's hand is kept still during the insertion of the needle and injection of the drugs. Once the needle or cannula is in the vein release the grip but do not let go until the patient is asleep because the needle can be dislodged during a sudden movement.

(b) *Inhalation induction*
This method is more commonly used in children than in adults. Usually an agent which produces anaesthesia rapidly is used. Cyclopropane used to be very popular for this purpose because it produced unconsciousness very rapidly but it has lost popularity due to its flammability. Nowadays nitrous oxide and halothane or enflurane are employed, increasing the concentration rapidly until consciousness is lost and then reducing it to a maintenance level.

(c) *Intramuscular induction*
Ketamine can be used intramuscularly to induce anaesthesia when vein puncture is difficult in, for example, children with severe burns.

(d) *Rectal administration*
Rectal thiopentone or methohexitone was widely used for children in the past. It popularity has waned because it has to be given beforehand,

administration was inconvenient, and the large doses used tended to cause a prolonged effect.

Intubation

Many anaesthetics can be administered with an inhalation agent given through a face mask (Figs 3.10 and 6.6). When relaxation of the muscles is required, as in abdominal surgery, when the lungs must be inflated during surgery in the open chest, when the anaesthetist needs to be away from the head as in ENT, neuro, head and neck and ophthalmic surgery and when the airway needs to be protected against potential aspiration of vomitus in emergency anaesthesia the trachea is usually intubated. This is commonly accomplished by paralysing the patient with muscle relaxants so that the jaw and larynx are relaxed. Less commonly intubation is performed under deep general anesthesia or with local anaesthesia applied to the mouth and larynx.

Intubation provides control of the airway when successfully performed but a number of potential problems exist. These include failed intubation, intubation of the oesophagus, kinking, or obstruction of the tube from debris or problems relating to the cuff. This may be compression of the lumen or an old cuff being distended over the end of the tube and occluding it. It is thus important to check ventilation of both sides of the chest by observation of chest movement and by listening with a stethoscope. This should also reveal when only one side is ventilating because the tube has been inserted beyond the trachea into a bronchus, a problem which is more common in infants because they have a short trachea.

Traumatic intubation, the use of too large a tube or excess pressure in the cuff may lead to postoperative laryngeal oedema, stridor due to partial airways obstruction and sore throat. The cuff pressure does not increase during nitrous oxide anaesthesia if the cuff is filled with the same gas as is being delivered to the patient. When air is used in the cuff the highly diffusible nitrous oxide enters the cuff expanding the gas volume and increasing the pressure in the cuff.

In children before puberty the circular cricoid cartilage is the narrowest part of the larynx. For this reason and because a cuff would take up too much of the cross-sectional area of the trachea cuffed tubes are usually not used until 6.5 mm or larger tubes are needed. The approximate size needed is age/4 + 4 mm internal diameter and usually a size bigger and one smaller are kept available. The larger size may be

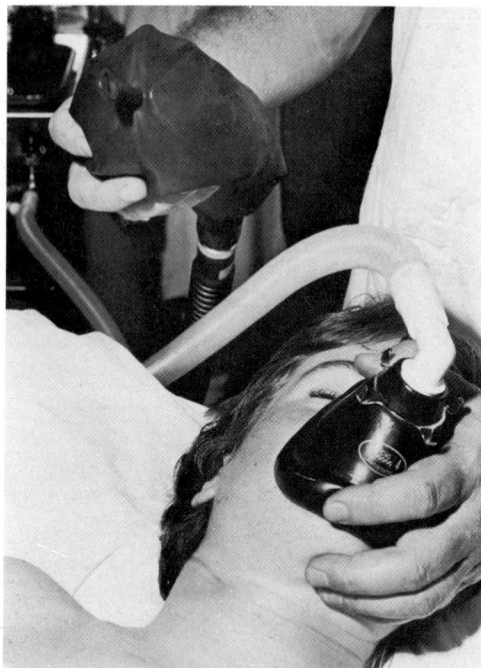

Fig. 6.6   The mask is held on the face by the thumb and index finger while the other fingers support the jaw. The patient can be ventilated by squeezing the bag with the other hand. The Bain circuit is shown.

appropriate with thin walled PVC tubes while the smaller internal diameter tubes are used when wall thickness is greater. A tube with minimum leak is the optimum size.

When muscle relaxants are used the anaesthetist has to ventilate the patient by the application of a face mask (Figs 6.6 and 6.7) and compressing the bag intermittently until the patient is sufficiently relaxed to intubate. The laryngoscope is usually held in the anaesthetist's left hand. It is inserted into the right side of the mouth so that the tongue is pushed to the left as the laryngoscope is advanced until the epiglottis and larynx come into view. The endotracheal tube is then passed with the right hand from the right corner of the mouth so that the vocal cords can be seen until the tube passes between them into the trachea (Fig. 6.8).

The assistant can be of great help during intubation, first, passing the laryngoscope to the anaesthetist so that he can take it in the left hand in

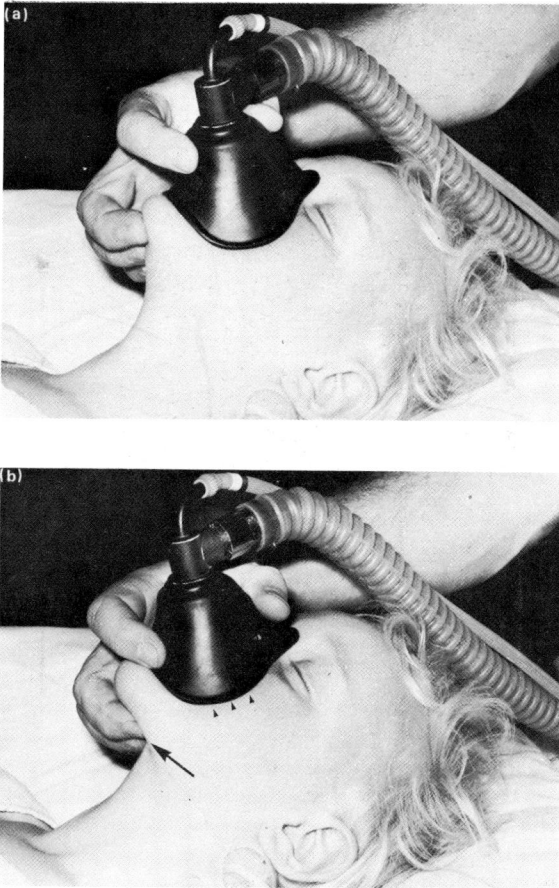

Fig. 6.7   (a) A Rendell Baker mask is held differently. It should be placed on the groove in the chin and the thumb and index finger are placed at the top of the mask as shown so that an airtight fit can be made. (b) This shows the wrong way to hold the mask. The thumb and index finger holding the mask lower down tends to make it splay and a gas leak develops. The other fingers are also compressing the tongue upwards in the midline instead of supporting the jaw (arrow).

the position ready to insert into the mouth (Fig. 6.9) and, secondly, handling the endotracheal tube to the anaesthetist (Fig. 6.10). If the larynx does not readily come into view some backward pressure on the

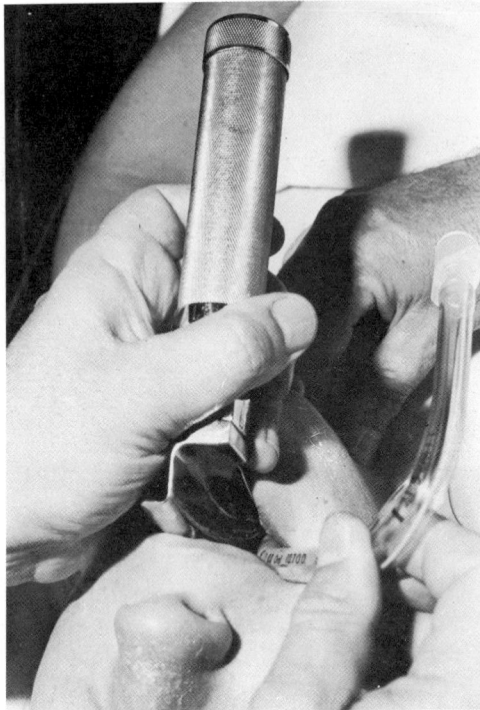

Fig. 6.8 Intubation. The laryngoscope is inserted so that the tongue is pushed to the left by the vertical part of the blade. The tube is passed from the right corner of the mouth so that it can be seen entering the larynx.

larynx may help to expose it (Fig. 6.11). The appropriate size and type of tube is passed with the appropriate connector, the circuit is then connected and the patient is ventilated and the tube is strapped or tied in place (Fig. 6.12). A supply of tape cut to appropriate lengths beforehand should be readily available. Sometimes when access to the face is difficult for the anaesthetist during the operation, as in neurosurgery, strapping the tube in can be an elaborate procedure to ensure that extubation or disconnection does not occur during the operation. If the head is to be covered by drapes or the patient to be lying face down the eyes are taped closed to prevent corneal damage. It is helpful to turn the lower outer corner of the tape inwards to facilitate removal at the end of the operation (Fig. 6.12). It may be necessary to use extra protective padding over

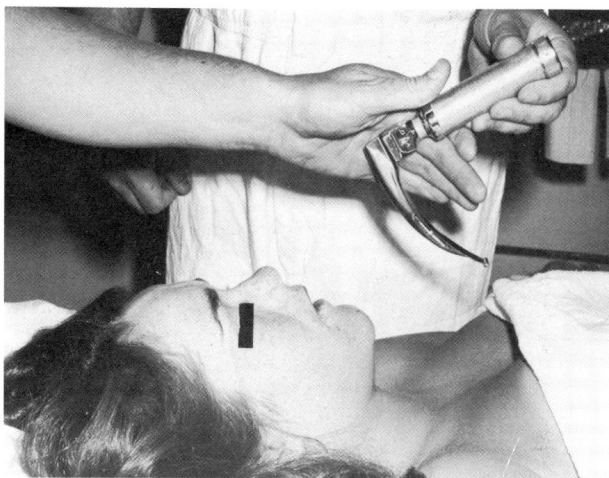

Fig. 6.9 The correct way to hand the laryngoscope to the anaesthetist so that it is open and can be taken by the anaesthetist in the position in which he will use it.

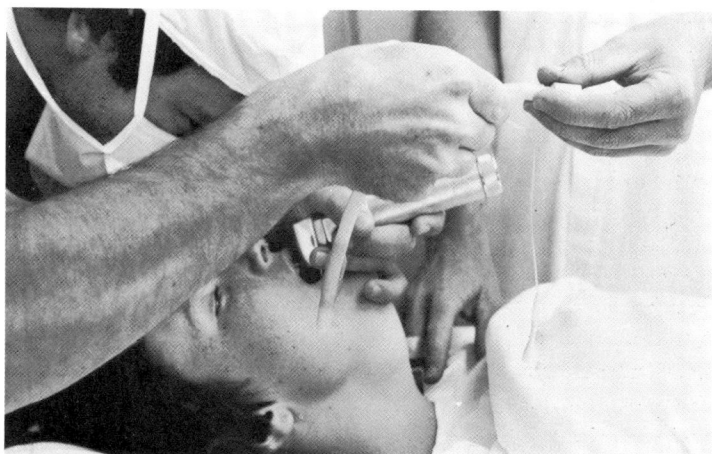

Fig. 6.10 The endotracheal tube is handed to the anaesthetist so that he can grasp it ready for insertion.

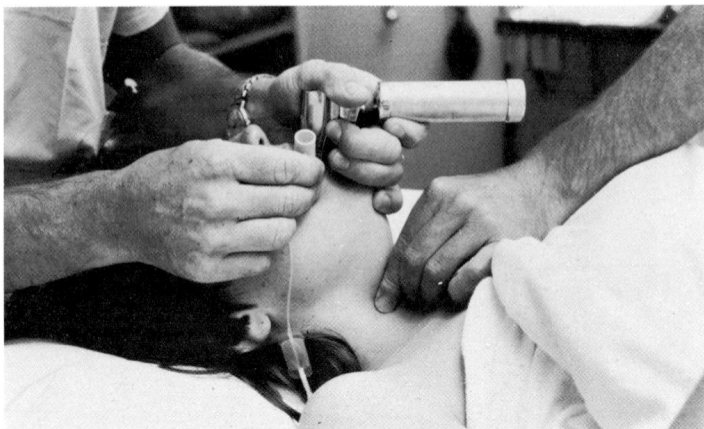

Fig. 6.11   Pressure backwards on the larynx by an assistant may help to bring the vocal cords more completely into view.

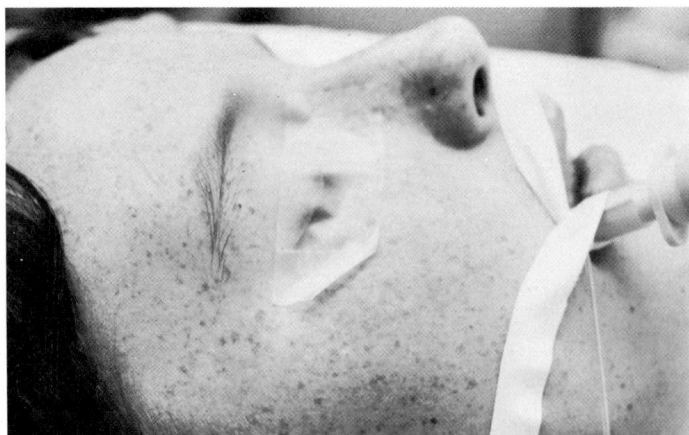

Fig. 6.12   If there is any danger of trauma to the cornea during procedures around the head and neck or if the eyelids tend to remain open they can be protected by taping the eyelids closed. Turning one corner in as shown facilitates removal at the end. The tube is usually anchored with tape.

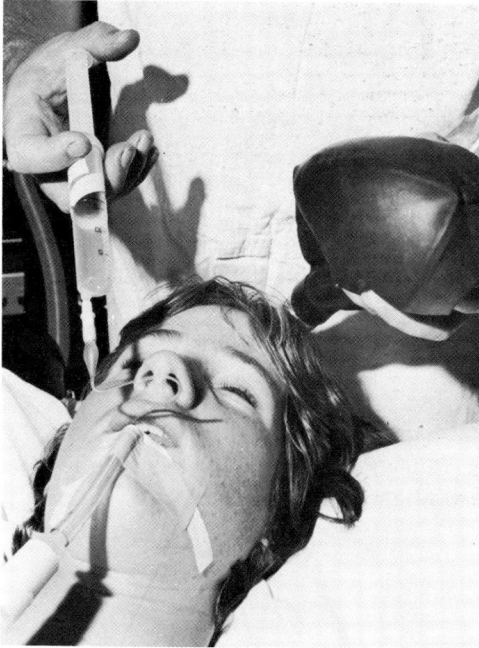

Fig. 6.13 When the tube is in place the cuff is inflated. While positive pressure is applied the cuff is blown up until the leak around the tube just disappears. It is preferable to use the gas being delivered from the anaesthetic machine to inflate the cuff to minimize pressure changes in the cuff during anaesthesia.

the eyes in neurosurgery when the face is placed in a head rest. The cuff is inflated as shown in Fig. 6.13.

Application of cricoid pressure

During emergency anaesthesia when it is suspected that the patient may have a 'full stomach' or if the patient has a hiatus hernia there is a danger of vomiting or regurgitation followed by aspiration of the regurgitated material into the trachea and lower airways. This can be very dangerous if lumps of food are inhaled because they cause respiratory obstruction, or if the material is very acid (pH below 2.5) because it causes an intense mucosal reaction with swelling and pulmonary oedema. This condition, called Mendelson's syndrome is particularly likely to occur in obstetrical emergencies and it is now common practice in obstetrics to give the mothers antacids during labour to raise the stomach pH and reduce the acidity.

A widely used method to prevent regurgitated material reaching the pharynx and being aspirated into the trachea is to apply cricoid pressure (Sellick's manoeuvre). The thumb and index finger are placed over the cricoid cartilage (immediately below the Adam's apple in the adult male) and pressed firmly back toward the vertebral column. The cricoid is a complete ring of cartilage while the tracheal cartilages are incomplete posteriorly. Backward pressure then compresses the oesophagus between the cricoid cartilage and vertebral body (Fig. 6.14). If the pressure is correctly applied the oesophagus is completely occluded and fluid cannot flow up into the pharynx.

In emergency anaesthesia a working sucker must always be readily available. The Yankauer sucker has an angle to facilitate pharyngeal suction. It is important to ensure the tip is screwed on tightly.

Posturing the patient

Patients are placed in a position to provide optimal surgical access. The site of operation and approach will therefore decide whether the patient

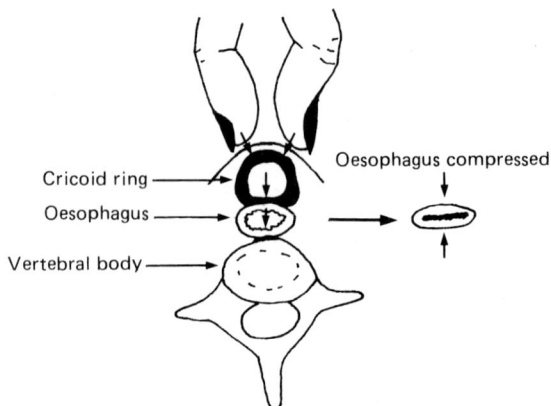

Fig. 6.14   The correct way to apply pressure to prevent regurgitation during induction is to place the thumb and index finger over the cricoid cartilage, which is a complete ring, and press firmly backwards thereby compressing the oesophagus on to the vertebrae. The cricoid cartilage is situated immediately below thyroid cartilage (Adam's apple).

is supine, prone, lateral, lithotomy or in head up position. The anaesthetist's assistant may play an important role in positioning the patient.

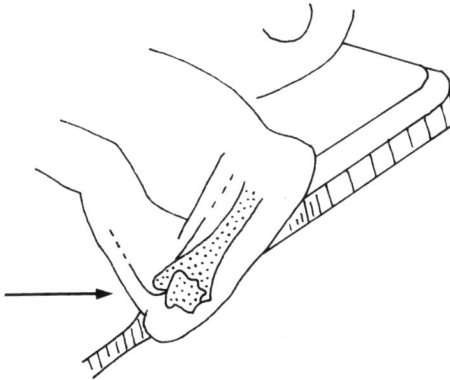

Fig. 6.15 The ulnar nerve can be compressed on the edge of the table if the elbow is allowed to hang over the edge. This may result in paraesthesia which can last for several months.

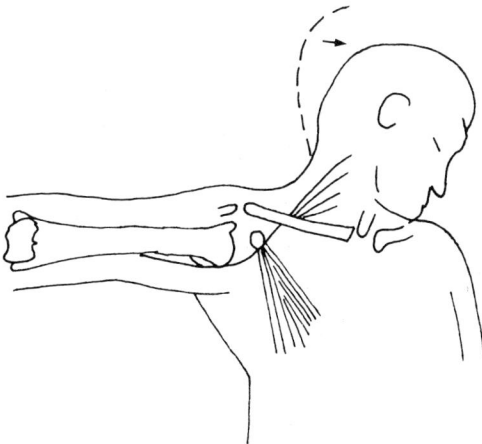

Fig. 6.16 Brachial plexus injury can result from stretching the nerves around fixed points. Rotation of the head away from a hyperextended arm can stretch the nerve. This can be aggravated further by rotating the arm. Brachial plexus injury can cause paraesthesia or weakness of the muscles supplied by the stretched nerves.

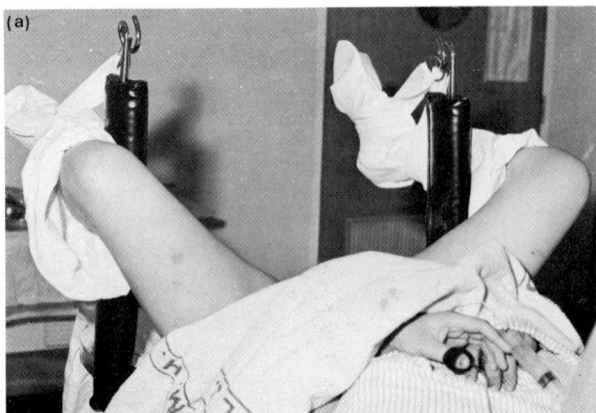

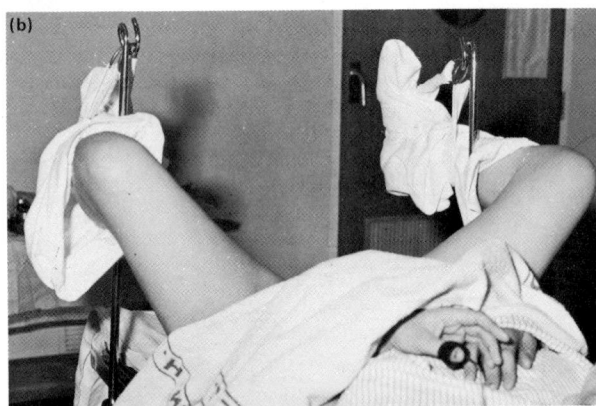

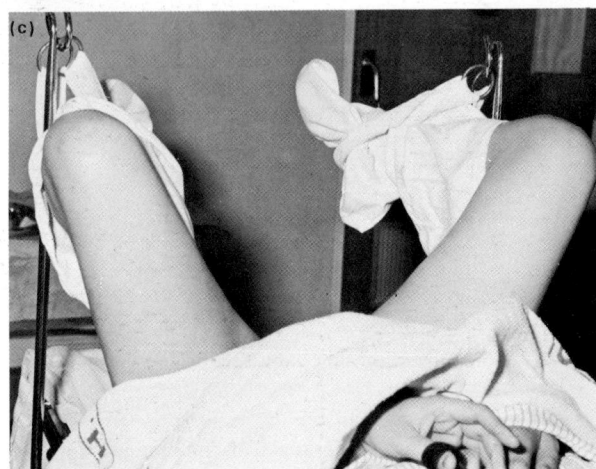

Fig. 6.17 (a) Legs in the correct position for lithotomy with padding to prevent compression, (b) in the incorrect position because there is no protective padding to prevent pressure on the saphenous nerve and (c) because the stirrup pole can compress the common peroneal (lateral popliteal) nerve as it courses round the head of the fibula. Note the pulse monitor applied to the left thumb.

The patient should be postured carefully during surgery. Pressure areas should be padded, especially in thin old people with poor circulation. It is important to avoid nerve damage. Bad positioning can result in stretching or compression of nerves leading to unpleasant and incapacitating neurological complications postoperatively. Examples include compression of the ulnar nerve when the elbow hangs over the edge of the table, (Fig. 6.15), stretching of the brachial plexus when the arm is hyperextended and the head is turned in the opposite direction (Fig. 6.16) or compression of the popliteal nerve (peroneal) when the legs are up in stirrups and there is no padding to prevent the nerve pressing on the leg supports (Fig. 6.17).

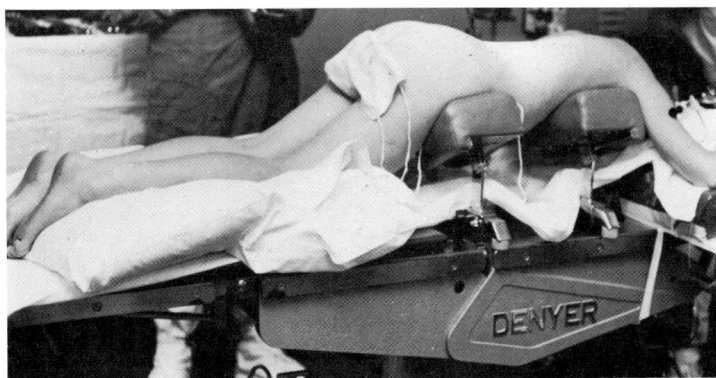

Fig. 6.18 A special frame used for back operations showing how the shoulders and hips are supported so that the abdomen can move freely with the descent of the diaphragm during respiration.

Patients in the prone (face down) position usually have their shoulders and hips supported so that the chest and abdomen can move freely during ventilation (Fig. 6.18). This prevents obstruction to venous return and congestion of veins which can cause undesirable bleeding during spinal surgery.

The lateral position is often used for renal surgery and for thoracotomy. A kidney bar raised under the patient helps to widen the distance between the iliac crest and lower ribs on the operative side improving access to the kidney. A bar or rolled towel may be placed under the chest to make the ribs spread apart wider when the chest is opened. It is preferable to place the intravenous infusion on the upper arm to ensure that it flows freely.

The lithotomy position is widely used in urology, gynaecology and perineal and anal surgery (e.g. hemorrhoidectomy). The legs are raised and held in stirrups. Care must be taken to prevent nerve compression (see above). The legs should be lowered gradually so that the sudden flow of blood back into the legs does not lead to hypotension. Often these procedures are done under spinal, epidural or caudal anaesthesia. Blockade of the sympathetic nerves to the lower body and limbs leads to vasodilatation and increases the capacitance of the circulation, hence decreasing venous return (see Chapter 4). If bleeding has occurred as well, but has been inadequately replaced because the circulation appeared adequate while the legs were raised, the patient may become hypotensive when the legs are lowered.

The head up or sitting position is sometimes used, especially in posterior fossa neurosurgery and during pneumoencephalography. Anaesthesia inhibits the cardiovascular reflexes which maintain blood pressure on rising from the horizontal. The result is that blood pressure and hence cerebral perfusion pressure may fall if care is not taken to raise the patient gradually and to give intravenous fluids to increase the blood volume thus compensating for the blood pooling in the lower part of the body. The legs may be bandaged or an antigravity suit can be used to reduce this pooling.

It is important, especially when moving to the sitting position, that someone controls the head so that neck injury and accidental extubation are avoided.

In the sitting or head up position there is a danger, especially in neurosurgery, of air entering an open vein in the head causing air embolism to the heart and pulmonary blood vessels. Hypotension and cardiac arrest can occur because flow of blood through the lungs is obstructed if much air enters.

In obstetrics a special problem called the supine hypotensive syndrome occurs if the patient lies supine. The gravid uterus compresses the inferior vena cava leading to a reduction of venous return and hypotension. This can be avoided by tilting the patient 15–30° to the left so that the uterus is not compressing the vena cava. Patients should be transported on their side.

The positioning of the anaesthetist

The anaesthetist occupies a position relative to the patient which allows free access for the surgeon, his assistant and scrub nurse to the operative site. For instance, the anaesthetist will be at the head of the table for abdominal, thoracic or lower limb surgery but is usually at the side of the patient during neuro, ENT and ophthalmic surgery (Fig. 6.19). He must be positioned so that he has access to the patient for monitoring and so that he can scan easily from the patient to the anesthetic machine and monitoring equipment.

The breathing circuit should be set up so that it lies in the appropriate direction and once the patient is postured it should be stabilized so

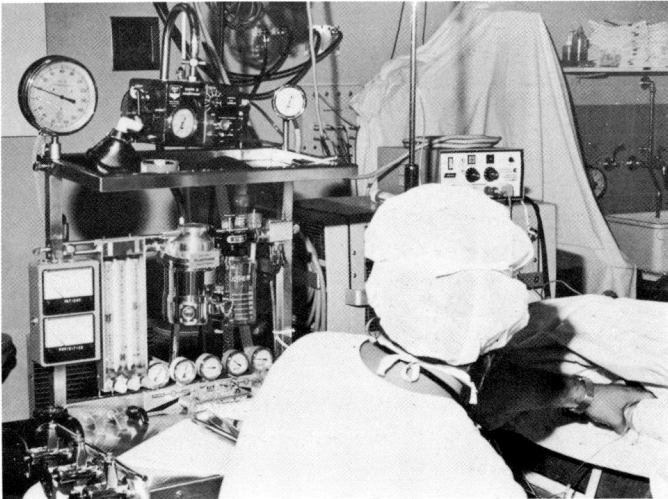

Fig. 6.19 The anaesthetist should be positioned so that he can observe the patient (pulse, colour and ventilation), the anaesthetic machine and monitoring devices within an arc requiring minimal movement. He should never have to turn his back to the patient to observe his machine or monitors.

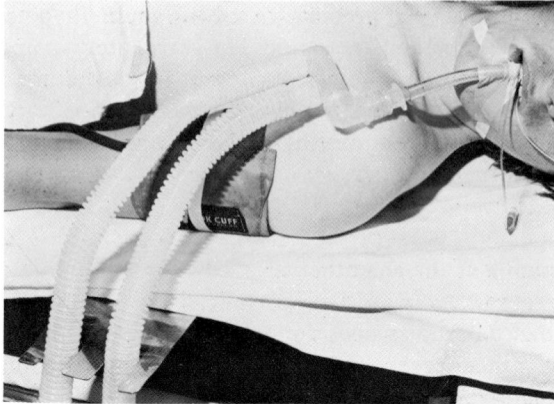

Fig. 6.20   The corrugated tubing can be stabilized in a clip to prevent traction on the tube which might lead to accidental extubation.

that it does not drag on the endotracheal tube causing accidental extubation (Figs 6.20 and 6.21).

An intravenous infusion is often inserted for the infusion of fluids or blood. The site chosen will often depend on the availability of suitable veins and the anaesthetist's preference but it should, if possible, be a site which is easily accessible during the operation.

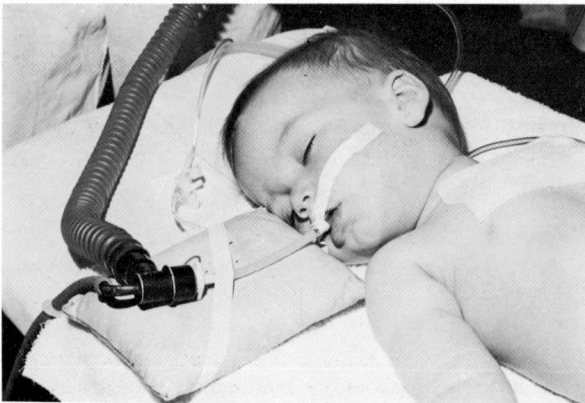

Fig. 6.21   The tube and connectors in small children can be stabilized by strapping them on a sandbag.

Application of diathermy and electrical equipment

When surgical diathermy is going to be used the indifferent electrode (diathermy plate) should be applied. It should be well covered with conductive jelly and closely applied to a large area of skin if burns are to be avoided. The connections between the plate and the machine should be checked to avoid faulty function. The patient's greatest protection when any electrical equipment is being attached is an intact earth wire in the mains power lead. Before connecting always examine the power lead carefully for (a) positive connection of all three wires at the power plug and (b) evidence of damage to the outer insulating sheath which might suggest interruption of any of the three wires. Do not connect any equipment which fails this inspection.

A fuller consideration of the principles of diathermy and the electrical hazards in theatre is included in Chapter 9.

Maintenance of general anaesthesia

The method used for the maintenance of general anaesthesia will depend on the nature and length of the operation. The patient may spontaneously breathe an inhalation anaesthetic such as halothane with nitrous oxide either from a mask or via an endotracheal tube which is usually inserted with the aid of a short period of muscle paralysis produced by suxamethonium. The alternative is to paralyse the patient throughout and maintain anaesthesia with nitrous oxide supplemented by an intravenous analgesic or a low concentration of inhalation anaesthetic. The patient is ventilated with a mechanical ventilator or manually by intermittent compression of the anaesthetic reservoir bag until the effects of the muscle relaxant have worn off or have been reversed, usually with neostigmine and atropine.

Regional anaesthesia

Regional (and local) anaesthesia can be used for surgery but is also increasingly being used for postoperative and post-traumatic pain relief. It is produced by injecting a local anaesthetic around a nerve, group of nerves or into the spinal canal either into the subarachnoid space (spinal anaesthetic) or extradural space (epidural anaesthetic) (Fig. 6.22). For

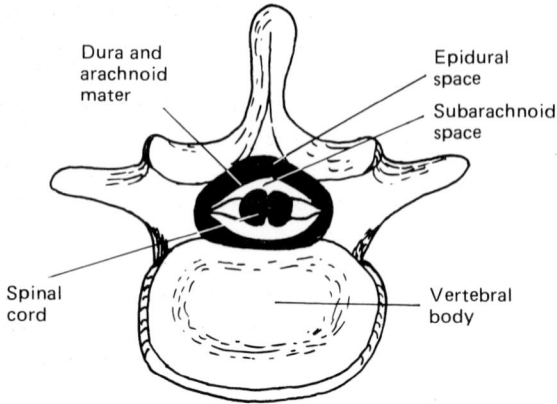

Fig. 6.22 Vertebra and spinal canal. In a spinal anaesthetic local anaesthetic is placed in the subarachnoid space usually at a level below the end of the spinal cord which normally reaches L1–2. Epidural anaesthesia is achieved by the injection of local anaesthetic into the epidural space where it blocks the nerves emerging through the dura.

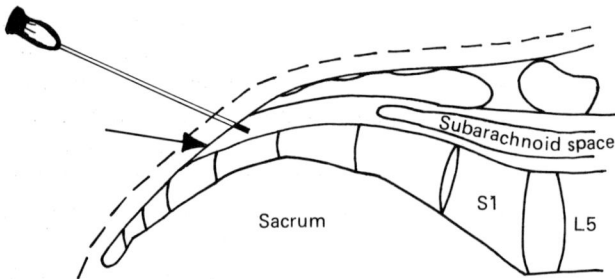

Fig. 6.23 The caudal canal is the lower end of the spinal canal as it passes through the sacrum. Caudal anaesthesia can be produced by injecting local anaesthetic through the membrane (arrowed) into the caudal extradural space where it blocks the lower spinal nerves.

caudal anaesthesia the local anaesthetic is injected through the sacral hiatus at the lower end of the spine into the epidural space (Fig. 6.23).

Spinal and epidural anaesthetics block several nerve roots on each side. The extent of the block is determined by the amount of local anaesthetic injected. The sympathetic nerves leaving the spinal cord are also blocked. These nerves exert vasoconstrictor tone on blood vessels so that when they are blocked the vessels in the affected area dilate and the blood pressure may drop. This factor is used to reduce blood loss, especially in gynaecological, perineal and penile surgery. Intravenous fluids may be needed to increase the blood volume if the fall in blood pressure is too great. It must be remembered that patients who have had spinal and epidural anaesthesia may have a lower than usual blood pressure in the recovery room.

Areas of the body can be anaesthetized by blocking the nerve supply to the region. A brachial plexus block performed by injection at the root of the neck or in the axilla provides anaesthesia for operations on the arm while a digital nerve block can be used for minor procedures on a finger.

An intravenous regional block can be used for procedures on the forearm such as manipulation of a fractured wrist. This involves applying two tourniquets on the upper arm and inserting a needle in a vein on the hand. The blood is then drained from the arm by compression with a bandage or by gravity and the proximal tourniquet is inflated above arterial pressure. About 40 ml of dilute local anaesthetic solution is then injected intravenously so that the nerves are blocked by vascular spread of the drug rather than by direct injection of the nerve. When the local anaesthetic has taken effect the distal tourniquet cuff is inflated above arterial pressure and the proximal one is deflated. This allows the area under the distal cuff to be anaesthetized otherwise the patient would have much discomfort. The tourniquets are used to allow the local anaesthetic to become fixed in the tissues and to prevent toxic blood levels of local anaesthetic reaching the general circulation. Usually this is avoided if the cuff is inflated for 20 minutes or longer.

Topical local anaesthesia is used mainly for procedures involving the nose, larynx, trachea and bronchi. Lignocaine (2-4%) is most commonly employed while cocaine (5-10%), which has a vasoconstrictor effect is often used in the nose.

(a) *Toxic effects of local anaesthetics*
These effects relate to the blood level attained and most commonly follow accidental intravascular injection. Circumoral tingling is often the first manifestation. The most serious effects are convulsions and cardiovascular depression due mainly to a direct depressant effect of the drug on the heart. Equipment and oxygen for resuscitation should always be readily available when regional blocks are performed.

(b) *Management of the patient*

Adult patients often tolerate operations under regional anaesthesia while remaining conscious but they are usually premedicated or given a tranquilizer such as diazepam. If the patient remains awake he or she should be given a full explanation beforehand of the procedure to take place. During the operation the anaesthetist should make sure that the patient is comfortable, converse with him or her if necessary and suppress inappropriate conversation amongst the staff in the theatre because the patient will hear it. It is more common in children to use local anaesthetic techniques in conjunction with light general anaesthesia.

Prior to performing the block it is important that the area to be injected is thoroughly prepared with antiseptic solution, that the syringes and needles are sterile and that the anaesthetist either wears gloves or thoroughly cleanses his hands using an antiseptic solution. An assistant can be very helpful during the performance of a block, especially a spinal or epidural, by helping to posture and hold the patient while the needle is inserted and the drug is injected.

Following regional and local anaesthesia it must be remembered that the analgesia may persist. This is often intentional so that the patient is pain free during the early postoperative period. Care must be taken to ensure that the insensitive areas are not injured by poor positioning or by plaster casts.

Conclusion of general anaesthesia

At the conclusion of the operation the action of the muscle relaxant is reversed if one has been used, the anaesthetic gases are turned off and the patient is ventilated gently with oxygen until breathing satisfactorily alone. When ventilation is adequate the pharynx should be sucked out carefully. Following nasal operations or adenoidectomy the neck should be flexed and the pharynx inspected with the laryngoscope to ensure no blood is trickling into the oropharynx. The patient is then extubated. If positive pressure is applied as the tube is removed the patient gives an explosive cough which clears any debris or blood from around the larynx as the patient is extubated.

The conclusion of anaesthesia can be a hazardous time for the patient. The anaesthetist should always have someone available to help in case a complication such as vomiting, laryngeal spasm or difficulty in ventilating the patient occurs. The patient should be turned on the side so that the tongue falls away and does not obstruct the airway and any

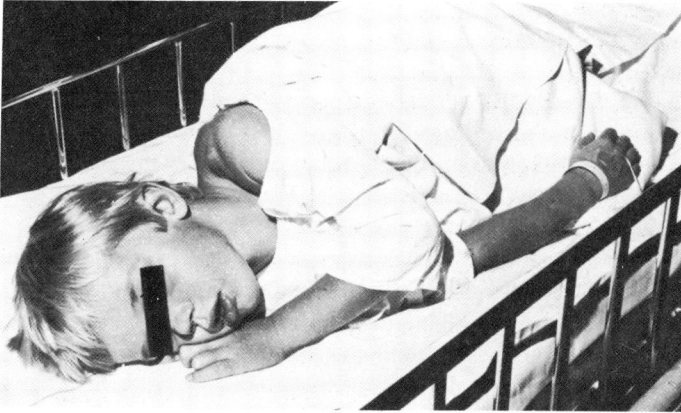

Fig. 6.24 Patient lying in the lateral position during recovery. The upper hand is placed under the jaw to prevent flexion of the neck which might lead to airway obstruction.

secretions drain out rather than being aspirated into the trachea. (Fig. 6.24).

If vomiting or regurgitation occur the patient should immediately be placed on the side (if not already in this position) with some head down tilt to allow drainage of vomitus out of the mouth. A sucker must always be ready for clearing any secretions, blood or vomitus from the mouth and pharynx.

If laryngeal spasm occurs the anaesthetist should apply continuous positive pressure with a mask with only oxygen flowing. Any brief break in the spasm then allows oxygen to enter the lungs. An assistant can be asked to open an ampoule of suxamethonium (a short acting relaxant) so that it can be drawn up and given intravenously. Its rapid onset of action may relieve the spasm more rapidly than waiting for the vocal cords to open spontaneously. Although the period of spasm is tense for the anaesthetist it usually breaks before severe hypoxia and cardiac arrest occur.

Chest drains

Following thoracic surgery any chest drains should be clamped near the patient before being moved. If the tubing is not clamped and the bottle is raised above the patient fluid can run back into the chest. It is also important to ensure that the tube from the chest is under water and that the fluid in the tube is swinging with respiration (Fig. 8.4).

Transfer to the recovery room

When the anaesthetist, at the conclusion of the anaesthetic, is satisfied that the patient is breathing adequately and is in a satisfactory condition he or she is moved on to a trolley or bed, preferably in the lateral position unless there is a reason to do otherwise. Trolleys should tilt easily so that the head can be lowered and should have sides so that the patient does not fall off. The patient is then transferred to the recovery room ensuring that a clear airway is maintained. Feeling the warm expired air with a hand held over the mouth and watching the patient's colour and chest movements are the ways in which the anaesthetist can easily monitor the adequacy of ventilation during transfer.

Care must be taken of intravenous lines and any other monitoring lines or chest drains to avoid dislodgement when the patient is moved. In some cases, particularly following major surgery, when the patient is in poor condition or where the patient has to be transferred long distances portable oxygen should be available for use during transport.

When the patient is being transferred to the recovery room the anaesthetist should always be accompanied by someone who can help to steer the trolley but, more importantly, can help if some complication occurs on the way. Some theatres are located some distance from the recovery room especially in large hospitals with many operating theatres and thus there is more time for problems to occur on the way.

CHAPTER 7

Intravenous fluids and blood transfusion

INTRAVENOUS FLUIDS DURING SURGERY   *Rate of administration. Choice of intravenous fluid.*
BLOOD TRANSFUSION   Blood groups. Blood grouping. Collection of blood. Blood components. Cross matching. Blood storage. Administration of blood. Complications of blood transfusion. Jehovah's witnesses.

Intravenous fluids and blood transfusion

Intravenous fluids during surgery

Patients having surgery often have some intravenous therapy. It may be started preoperatively especially if the patient is dehydrated or has lost blood (see Preoperative Resuscitation, Chapter 2). Operative fluid and blood requirements will depend on the nature and duration of surgery and the infusion may need to be continued into the postoperative period, especially when continuing losses are expected or when the patient is unlikely to be able to drink and eat for some time.

The basic physiology relating to blood and fluids is discussed in Chapter 4 (Blood and Body Fluids), and the equipment used is outlined in Chapter 6.

Fluid balance is achieved by the patient's fluid intake equalling losses from urine, sweating, insensible losses from skin, lungs and faeces and continuing pathological losses.

Rate of administration

During surgery a number of factors have to be considered when deciding how much fluid should be given. The daily maintenance requirement in an adult is 40 ml/kg/day. In children the requirements increase on a ml/kg/day basis as age decreases. Infants require 100 ml/kg/day although the amount is usually less during the first week of life.

The period of preoperative starvation and fluid deprivation should be taken into account. About 15 ml/kg could be given following an 8–10 hour fast. This can be increased in hot weather or if the patient is pyrexic because of increased losses through sweating.

The normal maintenance fluid requirements should continue to be given during the procedure. If preoperative rehydration is incomplete then additional fluid may need to be given rapidly and the induction of anaesthesia may need to be delayed. When the surgery involves opening the thorax or abdomen, especially when bowel is exposed, additional losses by evaporation can be expected.

Blood loss during surgery should be estimated. The simplest methods of measuring losses are to measure the volume in the sucker bottle (subtracting added fluid used by the surgeon if necessary) and weighing swabs and packs. An alternative is to wash out all swabs and packs in a tank and by measuring the haemoglobin of the solution and, knowing the volume of water contained, the volume of blood can be calculated, e.g.

$$1 \text{ g}/100 \text{ ml haemoglobin in 5 litres of water} = 50 \text{ g Hb}$$

$$\text{Patient's haemoglobin} = 12.5 \text{ gm}/100 \text{ ml}$$

$$\text{Blood loss} = (\text{total haemoglobin/patient's haemoglobin}) \times 100 \text{ ml} = 50/12.5 \times 100 = 400 \text{ ml}$$

When blood is lost there are fluid shifts in the body compartments to compensate. Often the amount of fluid needed to bring the patient back to normal is greater than might be expected. This is due to movement of fluid into tissues traumatized either by injury or the surgical procedure.

When significant blood loss or blood volume deficit is present central venous pressure monitoring is a useful guide during replacement. With blood loss the level falls and as it is replaced the level will rise towards normal. Over transfusion will cause an elevation in central venous pressure. Clinical signs of pulse and blood pressure can be used as well in the assessment — the pulse rises as blood volume decreases (see Cardio-vascular System, Chapter 4). It may be apparent during surgery that further blood or fluid losses can be expected. The infusion will then have to be maintained longer and this factor will have to be taken into consideration.

It can be seen that many factors influence the rate at which the intravenous infusion is run during an operation. It is often run rapidly during the first hour while maintenance deficits are made up.

It is most important to keep an accurate fluid balance chart.

Choice of fluid

There is a choice of fluids which can be used. Ideally the fluid should be isotonic with blood. Dextrose solutions provide calories although not usually enough for daily requirements. Five percent dextrose contains 50 g/litre which provides 200 calories. Excessive use of 5% dextrose without any electrolytes will lead to dilutional hyponatraemia (low sodium in the plasma). When maintenance fluids are required the solution should contain some sodium chloride as these are the major plasma ions (see Body Fluid, Chapter 4). Other electrolytes such as potassium are sometimes added in much lower concentrations to simulate normal plasma levels.

Hartmann's solution contains sodium, potassium, calcium, chloride and lactate. There are other similar solutions of the electrolytes approaching that of plasma. They are often used as maintenance fluids during surgery before significant blood loss has occurred.

Blood transfusion

The body can easily compensate for the loss of 500 ml or 10% of the blood volume. The transfusion of blood is not usually commenced until it is likely that two or more units of blood (1 litre +) will need to be given.

If substantial blood loss may occur during the operation blood is taken from the patient beforehand for grouping and an appropriate amount of blood is cross matched for possible transfusion during and after the operation.

Blood groups

There are at least 15 major well defined blood groups but only the A, B, O and the Rh systems are of major clinical importance in blood transfusion. Other groups are of less importance because they are less antigenic or the antibodies directed against them only develop after multiple transfusions.

When blood is grouped for the ABO system the red cells will have either group A antigen, group B antigen, both antigens (group AB) or none of the antigens (group O). The body produces antibodies directed against the ABO group antigens not present on the red cells. Thus a group A person has anti-B, group B people have anti-A, group O people have both anti-A and anti-B and group AB individuals have neither antibody in their plasma.

The Rh system is more complicated. There are three pairs of antigens named C and c, D and d, E and e. Each person has one or both of each pair. About 85% of the population has D antigen (in addition to the other Rh antigens) and are referred to as Rh positive. The remainder have dd and are called Rh negative. Antibodies to Rh blood group antigens do not occur naturally but are produced following transfusion. Thus an Rh negative person will produce anti-D antibodies following transfusion with Rh positive blood.

Blood grouping

It is of extreme importance when blood is taken for grouping and cross matching that the sample is labelled immediately with the patient's name and hospital unit number. The tube may be labelled just before the blood is drawn from the patient.

The patient's blood group is determined by adding the patient's washed red cells to separate samples of serum containing anti-A, and anti-B, for the ABO grouping and anti-D antibodies for the Rh grouping. If clumping occurs the cells have those antigens on the red cells. Thus group AB Rh positive will have clumping of cells with all three sera, while A Rh negative will clump only with anti-A antibodies. Group O Rh negative will not clump with any antibodies. Group O Rh negative can be given to patients in an extreme emergency if the blood group of the patient is not known because the patient's plasma will not react with the donor cells when transfused. It is, however, safer to give the patient's own blood group (this can be determined quickly) or wait until the blood is crossmatched.

Collection of blood

Blood is usually donated by healthy people who are not anaemic between the ages of 18 and 65 years. Donor blood is not collected from people who have had infections such as hepatitis A or B (Australian antigen), malaria or syphilis, or people who are taking medication. Tests are usually conducted on all donors to ensure that they are not carrying any of these diseases at the time of donation.

The blood is collected into plastic bags containing either acid citrate dextrose (ACD) or citrate phosphate dextrose (CPD) which prevent the blood clotting by inactivating calcium which is essential in normal clotting. Occasionally fresh blood is needed. This can be anticoagulated with heparin, but it cannot be stored for the long periods permitted with ACD (21 days) and CPD (28 days) blood.

Blood components

Cells from donor blood are now frequently separated from the plasma. Packed red cells may be supplied instead of whole blood from patients undergoing surgery. An electrolyte solution such as Hartmanns or Ringer's lactate is commonly added to reduce the haematocrit and hence the viscosity of the blood before transfusion. The components prepared from the separated plasma include the following:

Stable plasma protein solution (SPPS) which is an osmotically active plasma volume expander.

Concentrated albumin (25%) which can be used in patients with hypo-proteinaemia. These people develop oedema due to the lack of protein and reduction of osmotic pressure in the plasma (see Fig. 2.1).

Albumin (5%) which is less commonly used for plasma volume expansion.

Fresh frozen plasma which contains the clotting factors. This is used when there is a coagulation defect and the patient's blood does not clot. When thawing prior to administration it should not be warmed over 37°C.

Platelets can be separated for administration in thrombocytopenia or when the platelets do not function normally — this can occur following salicylate ingestion. Platelet preparations should not be refrigerated.

Factor VIII (AGH) and cryoprecipitate which are used in the treatment of haemophilia when bleeding occurs or prophylactically before surgery or dental extractions.

Cross matching

This involves exposure of the red cells to be transfused into the patient to antibodies which the patient has or may have developed in his own serum. The techniques are designed to detect these antibodies.

The patient's blood group is determined and his or her serum is mixed with cells from the pilot tubes attached to bags of blood of the same group. If they are compatible no clumping occurs. This unit then has a label attached with the proposed recipients name and unit number and the number of the unit of blood so that all can be checked before transfusion is started.

Blood storage

Blood is stored in special refrigerators at 4°C. If blood is left out for more than an hour without administering it to the patient it should not be transfused but returned to the blood bank. The plasma may then be used for separation into some of the components.

During storage potassium from the cells leaks out into the plasma so that after 2–3 weeks high levels of potassium are present. This usually equilibrates back into the cells following transfusion but if very rapid transfusion is necessary dangerous levels of serum potassium may be reached and cardiac arrest can occur. If massive transfusion is necessary it is preferable to use recently collected blood.

ACD blood becomes increasingly acidotic on storage due to the formation of lactate. Rapid transfusion of old blood can cause an acidosis which may have a depressant effect on myocardial contractility, but usually the acidosis is transient. Eventually, as perfusion improves, the citrate is metabolized to bicarbonate and following massive transfusion an alkalosis may develop.

ACD and CPD inactivate calcium in the blood. Under normal rates of transfusion the liver can metabolize these and calcium can be mobilized so that normal levels are maintained. When blood is very rapidly transfused (500 ml in 5 minutes or half the blood volume in 1 hour) there is not always time for this to happen and, if the patient is hypotensive, the liver may not be well perfused so that serum calcium levels fall. This affects clotting and also reduces myocardial contractility, so that it is wise under these circumstances to give additional calcium (5 ml 10% calcium gluconate for each unit of blood). This should not be injected into the blood container as clotting may occur. The calcium will also counteract the adverse effects of hyperkalaemia.

Administration of blood

The equipment used is discussed in Chapter 6. The unit of blood must be carefully checked to ensure that it is for the correct patient. The name and unit number must be the same on the patient's identification band, history, crossmatch slip and the label on the unit of blood. Incompatible transfusions are far more frequently due to clerical mistakes than to crossmatching errors. An incompatible transfusion has resulted from confusion due to mixing of the unit numbers of two patients on the same ward with the same name having the same operation on the same day.

When large volumes are being given and blood is transfused rapidly it is advisable to warm the blood before administration. This prevents rapid cooling of the heart, the development of arrhythmias and cardiac arrest. It is passed through coils in a blood warmer containing warm water. The blood temperature should not exceed body temperature. These precautions are not essential with the majority of transfusions.

Complications of blood transfusion

1 Infection is minimized by keeping the whole infusion system closed and by ensuring that the cannula is inserted without contamination. The correct handling of the blood, storing it at 4°C and testing the donors as described all reduce the chance of infection. Contamination of the blood after collection is usually with gram negative organisms. Haemolysis occurs and the plasma becomes discoloured.
2 Pyrogenic reactions. The blood may contain substances which cause a mild reaction in the patient usually resulting in a rise in temperature and tachycardia.
3 Incompatible transfusion may cause tachycardia, hypotension and signs of haemolysis. Bleeding is aggravated due to the development of disseminated intravascular coagulation in which the normal clotting factors and platelets are used up.
4 The problems of hyperkalaemia, acidosis and hypocalcaemia associated with massive transfusion have already been discussed.
5 Hypothermia and rapid cooling of the heart may increase myocardial irritability. Ventricular fibrillation can occur when body temperature reaches 28–29°C in adults and 26–27°C in small children. There is a real danger of cardiac arrest if cold blood is given too fast. The increased myocardial irritability may be aggravated by hyperkalaemia and hypocalcaemia.
6 Allergic reactions are most likely in patients who have had multiple transfusions, but may occur in people with an atopic tendency. The reactions vary in intensity from pyrexia to urticaria and rarely anaphylaxis where the patient may become acutely hypotensive or develop bronchospasm. Reactions in allergic people can be minimized by giving

an antihistamine such as chlorpheniramine 10 mg intramuscularly or intravenously before starting the transfusion.

Jehovah's Witnesses

People belonging to this religious group believe that there is a Biblical basis for their view that blood transfusion is not allowed. This causes a very difficult moral problem in the event of life threatening blood loss. Most doctors respect their view and methods have been devised to manage these patients without blood transfusion for major surgery including open heart surgery. In some cases some of the patient's blood is drawn off at the beginning and replaced with electrolyte solution or plasma volume expander (but not those derived from blood) and the patient's own blood is returned at the end of operation. This technique is called haemodilution. Another alternative is to vasodilate the patient thereby lowering the blood pressure so that less bleeding occurs and at the same time giving crystalloid fluids (electrolyte solutions) to increase the blood volume and temporarily haemodilute the blood. Very occasionally legal methods are invoked in young children to transfuse these patients if their life is in danger from blood loss.

CHAPTER 8

Recovery room

Equipment. Drugs and fluids. Handing over the patient. Observations, interpretation of signs and management. Postoperative vomiting. Oxygen therapy. Postoperative analgesia. Special care. Staffing and responsibility. Return to the ward.

The postoperative recovery room provides a site for continuing care of the patient at a less intensive level than in theatre but more intensive than in the normal ward. Patients are cared for there until they become fully conscious and their condition is stable. This usually means that they stay for about half to one hour but it may be for longer if recovery is delayed, complications occur, or after major surgery. This chapter will not consider complicated postoperative care, such as following cardiac surgery which is normally undertaken in a specialized intensive care unit.

Equipment

The recovery room should be equipped with oxygen and suction outlets for each bed and power points in case electronic monitoring devices or a defibrillator are needed. There should be a variety of sizes of anaesthetic masks and airways, bags and equipment for ventilation. Most recovery rooms have a ventilator available in case prolonged postoperative ventilation is necessary. In many hospitals the patient is transferred to the intensive care unit if this becomes necessary. Laryngoscopes and a set of endotracheal tubes should be available in case a patient requires intubation.

Drugs and fluids

A variety of intravenous fluids, giving sets and cannulae must be available. Resuscitation drugs (listed in Table 8.1), syringes and needles must be conveniently located and accessible for immediate use if required. Other drugs which often have to be given in the recovery room and should be available are analgesics and antibiotics, antidotes such as neostigmine and atropine for residual muscle paralysis, naloxone for respiratory depression and physostigmine for postoperative confusion. The action of these drugs is explained in more detail in Chapter 5. Some drugs used in the treatment of medical conditions may also be kept to be readily available if needed. Steroids may be used to minimize cerebral oedema in neurosurgical patients, to increase the stress response in patients who have had steroid treatment and whose adrenal function is suppressed, in shock and in the treatment of bronchospasm if bronchodilators are unsuccessful.

Table 8.1 Resuscitation drugs.

Drug	Use
Adrenaline	Myocardial stimulant and bronchodilator
Isoprenaline	
Sodium bicarbonate	Correction of metabolic acidosis
Calcium gluconate or chloride	Increases myocardial contractility especially in presence of hyperkalaemia
Atropine	To increase heart rate
Glucose 50%	Hypoglycaemia
Potassium chloride	To correct deficits and treat digoxin toxicity
Magnesium chloride	
Lignocaine	Used as an antiarrhythmic sometimes following defibrillation if the rhythm is unstable. (Also a local anaesthetic)

Handing over the patient

When the patient comes to the recovery room the anaesthetist hands over the responsibility for the continuing observation to a nurse. It is important that he or she should be told the patient's name, the operation and site, the type of anaesthetic given, about any problems that occurred or might be expected and whether any analgesics have been given.

Instructions regarding intravenous fluids or blood should be given and the postoperative orders should be completed. The latter is often done by the surgeon. The anaesthetist and nurse should check the patient's ventilation and circulation and the anaesthetist should not leave until both are satisfied with the patient's condition. The nurse should have a completed anaesthetic record to refer to should any problems occur. The operative site, dressing and drains should be observed when the patient is received. Plaster casts should be checked to ensure that they are not causing circulatory obstruction to limbs or pressure areas.

Observations, interpretation of signs and management

Observations carried out should be a continuation of those undertaken in the operating theatre — ventilation, pulse, blood pressure, colour and temperature. In neurosurgical patients conscious state, pupil size and reactivity are also observed.

This section aims to highlight important points. The reader should consult Chapter 4 for a more detailed discussion explaining the significant physiological changes in relation to monitoring.

(a) *Ventilation*
This is assessed by observation of colour, chest movement and by feeling the flow of warm expired air on the hand placed over the patient's mouth and nose (Fig. 8.1). In addition volume can be measured with a respirometer and blood gases (Pa,CO_2 and Pa,O_2) can be measured.

Inadequate ventilation may be due to airway obstruction or to hypoventilation most commonly caused in the postoperative period by drug depression or inadequate reversal of muscle relaxants. In either case the patient may eventually become cyanosed, hypoxic (low Pa,O_2) and develop carbon dioxide retention (increased Pa,CO_2). *Airway obstruction* can present with noisy breathing caused by secretions or blood, or with stridor associated with laryngeal oedema, upper airway narrowing or laryngeal spasm. Tracheal tug (Fig. 4.2), with sternal and rib retraction can occur when the inflow of air during inspiration is reduced due to airway obstruction and a greater negative intrathoracic pressure is generated in the chest.

The commonest cause of respiratory obstruction in unconscious patients is the tongue falling back into the pharynx. This can be relieved by pulling the jaw forward preferably with the mouth open, extending the head and placing the patient on the side. Sometimes the patient will

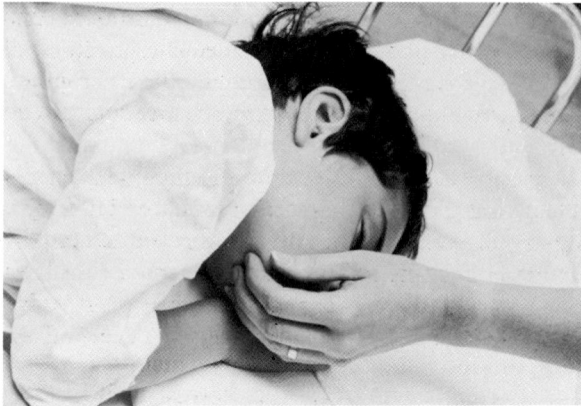

Fig. 8.1 Feeling for the warm expired breath is one of the ways of monitoring ventilation. Chest movements and colour should also be observed. The patient is shown in the lateral recovery position.

tolerate an oral airway especially when still unconscious. Any secretions or blood should be sucked out of the pharynx.

Laryngeal stridor can be alarming. Sometimes the anaesthetist will warn the nurses that this may occur, especially after bronchoscopy or laryngoscopy, and particularly in children. Another cause, also more common in children, occurs in patients who are returned to the recovery room still partially anaesthetized with halothane or enflurane. These agents sometimes cause stridor or laryngeal spasm at a light plane of anaesthesia. If stridor is worsening and other signs or respiratory obstruction occur help should be sought, preferably from the anaesthetist who gave the anaesthetic if he is available. In the meantime someone should administer oxygen by mask and the emergency drug and intubation trolley or equipment should be brought to the bedside.

If difficulty in relieving the obstruction and maintaining an adequate airway continues laryngoscopy and intubation may be necessary.

A special situation exists following thyroid surgery where haemorrhage into the operative site may cause tracheal compression. This can be relieved by prompt reopening of the wound. These patients may also have cord palsy if the recurrent laryngeal nerve is damaged during surgery.

Hypoventilation may result from inadequate reversal of muscle relaxants or from depression due to opiates or from residual effects of the anaesthetic.

Partially paralysed patients have incoordinate, jerky breathing, floppy limbs and do not expand their chest adequately. They will usually improve with additional doses of neostigmine with atropine. Positive pressure ventilation with a mask should be continued until ventilation is adequate.

Drug depression usually causes slow and shallow breathing. If it is suspected that it is due to opiates (morphine and similar drugs) it can be reversed with naloxone. This drug should be given in small increments because it reverses both the respiratory depressant and analgesic effects and if too much is given the patient may suffer pain. It is short acting (half an hour) so that a further dose may be needed if respiratory depression recurs.

Recovery from deep anaesthesia takes time and the patient should be nursed on the side until awake.

Some patients have reduced respiratory reserve preoperatively. These include patients with lung disease, muscular dystrophies, some neurological disease and severe kyphoscoliosis. These patients require special care during anaesthesia and careful observation in the recovery room. If there is any doubt about the airway or ventilation an anaesthetist should be called. A bag and mask, laryngoscope, tubes, muscle relaxant (suxamethonium) and suction should be on hand in case assisted ventilation or intubation is necessary.

The commonest complications in the recovery room are problems with ventilation and, if untreated, these can go on to hypoxia and cardiac arrest.

(b) *Pulse*

A steadily rising pulse is usually significant. It may be associated with bleeding when the pulse will become thready or softer because less blood is pumped by the heart with each beat. A bounding, fast pulse is usually associated with increased sympathetic system activity (adrenaline response) resulting from a rising Pa,co_2 due to hypoventilation or to pain.

Bradycardia associated with a rising blood pressure may indicate rising intracranial pressure in patients with head injuries or following intracranial operations. Marked slowing of the pulse in infants and small children is associated with hypoxia.

An irregular pulse is usually associated with heart disease but is occasionally due to the action of drugs. In young people a physiological variation in heart rate associated with respiration is called sinus arrhythmia and is of no pathological significance.

(c) *Blood pressure*

Hypotension may result from the following:

1 Decreased blood volume due to bleeding or inadequate replacement of blood or fluid losses.

2 A decrease in cardiac output caused by myocardial disease or drug induced myocardial depression.

3 Sometimes when the blood vessels are dilated and the peripheral resistance is reduced. In the recovery room this most commonly follows spinal and epidural anaesthesia.

The operative site, wound, or arterial pucture site following angiography should be observed for bleeding. Hypotension due to blood loss is associated with a rising pulse and pallor of the skin and mucous membranes. If the patient becomes hypotensive an intravenous infusion should be set up and blood may need to be cross matched. Local pressure should be applied if this will control the bleeding.

Vasodilatation with reduction of peripheral resistance can result from the use of vasodilating drugs or with epidural or spinal anaesthesia where sympathetic vasoconstrictor nerves are blocked. Blood pressure is lowered but because cardiac output is usually maintained the hands and feet will be well perfused and feel warm. If the blood pressure is too low and cardiac output decreases additional intravenous fluids are given to raise central venous pressure and improve ventricular filling. Cardiac output should then increase. If cardiac output is depressed significantly from inadequate blood volume or myocardial dysfunction the heart sounds will be softer when listened to with a stethoscope, the circulation to the hands and feet may be sluggish so that capillary refill following pressure on a finger or toe will be slow and the periphery may feel cold and have a pale bluish tinge.

Febrile patients may have peripheral vasodilatation to facilitate heat loss but they also have an increased cardiac output and a bounding pulse.

Faithful recording of pulse and blood pressure is useless if no action is taken when significant changes occur. The surgeon or anaesthetist looking after the patient should be informed.

(d) *Temperature*

The patient's temperature should be recorded on return to the recovery room. There is a tendency for patients to cool during anaesthesia due to depression of the temperature regulating centre in the hypothalamus, decreased muscle tone, peripheral vasodilatation especially with drugs such as halothane, and increased heat loss when body cavities are opened. Cold patients are peripherally vasoconstricted which makes them look pale and, when the peripheral circulation is sluggish, peripheral cyanosis may develop.

The consequences of cooling, which is especially common in infants and children, are delayed recovery from anaesthesia and increased oxygen consumption and metabolic rate associated with increased heat production and shivering.

When patients are cold on return to the recovery room they may be warmed up to normal temperature before returning to the ward. They should be kept warm with blankets and can be actively warmed with an electric or warm water circulating blanket or by using 'space blankets' which reflect the patients radiated heat back to them. These are very effective and eliminate the potential hazard of burns when other active means of warming are used. Following anaesthesia with halothane or trilene patients are often very rigid and may shiver. This is more common when the temperature is low but can occur in normothermic individuals.

An elevation of temperature is uncommon following anaesthesia but may be due to infection, a reaction to blood transfusion, over enthusiastic application of methods to prevent cooling or in association with some rare diseases. Patients with malignant hyperpyrexia develop very high temperatures but this usually occurs during anaesthesia. Immediate treatment with active cooling, oxygenation and correction of acidosis is essential if a fatal outcome is to be avoided (see Malignant Hyperpyrexia, Chapter 4).

(e) *Conscious state and pupillary reactions*
A deterioration in conscious state or responsiveness to verbal or physical stimuli should be cause to review the patient's condition. It should not be confused with the patient going back to sleep. It is a very important sign in neurosurgical patients or following major trauma especially if the head is injured.

Alterations in the size of the pupils, particularly if one dilates more than the other, and their responsiveness to light are important following neurosurgery (see Chapter 4). The surgeon should be notified immediately.

(f) *Other patient reactions*
Patients who thrash around may be in pain, hypoxic, disorientated or have a distended bladder. It is important to differentiate pain, which can be treated with analgesics, from hypoxia, where a clear airway, oxygen

and possibly ventilation are required, from disorientation. The latter may settle with intravenous physostigmine especially when hyoscine has been used. A full bladder can be managed by getting the patient to void if possible, expressing the bladder or occasionally a catheter will need to be inserted. Overdistension can lead to bladder dysfunction.

Distressed and frightened children can be soothed by kind handling by the recovery room staff or by the presence of a parent if they are allowed into the recovery room. Sometimes infants cry because of hunger.

Postoperative vomiting

This is common following anaesthesia and occurs in 10-50% of patients. Many factors influence the incidence including age, sex and type of anaesthetic and the operation. In the recovery room vomiting is hazardous if the patient's laryngeal reflexes have not returned because aspiration into the trachea and bronchi may cause respiratory obstruction. If the gastric contents are very acid, aspiration results in a severe chemical reaction causing pulmonary oedema. This is known as Mendelson's syndrome and occurs most commonly in obstetric anaesthesia. In some hospitals antacids are given preoperatively to reduce the likelihood of this occurrence.

The danger of inhalation of gastric contents is reduced if the patient is placed on the side and the trolley tilted head down. Suction equipment should be ready for use at all times to clear the airway if vomiting occurs.

Patients who have a fractured jaw or who have had mandibular surgery pose a special problem if their jaws have been fixed together with wires or hooks with elastic bands. A pair of wire cutters or scissors must always be at the bedside to cut the wires if the patient vomits so that the pharynx can be cleared.

Oxygen therapy

In some recovery rooms oxygen is administered routinely to all patients recovering from anaesthesia while in others it is only given following prolonged anaesthesia or to patients considered to be at risk from hypoxia.

The oxygen tension in the blood (Pa,o_2) immediately following anaesthesia is commonly lower than usual. Often the decrease in oxygen tension is not clinically significant, especially in young, healthy patients but in older patients, particularly those with respiratory or cardiovascular disease hypoxia may occur which may cause myocardial ischaemia and decreased cardiac utput.

The short term administration of additional oxygen is harmless and is likely to be beneficial during recovery from anaesthesia in most patients. Care must be taken not to give excessive oxygen to patients with emphysema, who are dependent on a hypoxic drive to breathe because they have become insensitive to a chronically elevated Pa,co_2, and to premature infants, who can develop retrolental fibroplasia and visual damage when exposed to high oxygen concentrations for prolonged periods.

Oxygen should preferably be administered by a light plastic mask, but nasal prongs or nasal catheter are also used. Gastric distension and mucosal damage are potential hazards with a catheter.

A portable oxygen supply should be available for the transport of patients who have to be transferred to wards with additional oxygen.

Postoperative analgesia

Most surgical procedures are associated with some postoperative pain or discomfort. The amount of analgesia required will depend on the operation, the patient's condition and response to pain. Traditionally opiates such as morphine and pethidine have been used by 3–4 hourly intramuscular injections followed later by milder analgesics as the pain subsides. Sometimes an analgesic given with the premedication or during surgery is sufficient to provide the initial postoperative analgesia.

The problem with intermittent intramuscular analgesic administration is that a larger than necessary dose is needed to maintain an effective blood level for long enough. If the next injection is not given soon enough the blood level drops so that the patient begins to feel pain again. Recently the use of intravenous administration by infusion has been developed. A loading dose is given to achieve a therapeutic blood level and then the infusion rate is set to keep the patient pain free. Figure 8.2 illustrates these different blood level patterns. The response of the patient is necessarily involved in establishing the appropriate rate. Using this method the peaks and troughs in blood level are avoided, less total dose of analgesic is needed and hence the incidence of vomiting and respiratory depression is reduced.

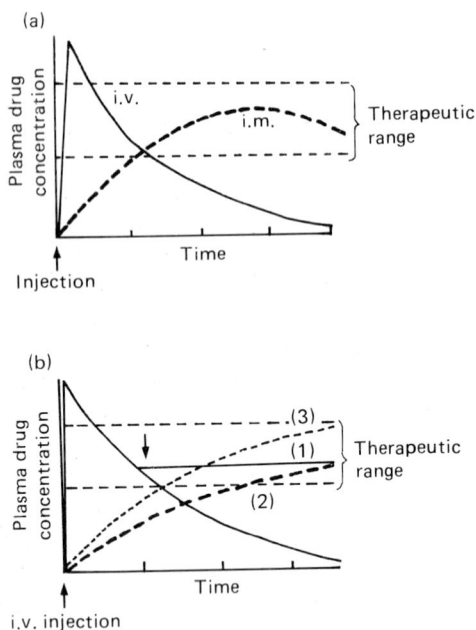

Fig. 8.2 (a) An intravenous bolus of drug causes a rapid rise in plasma concentration and a fairly rapid decline as the drug is redistributed to the tissues. The plasma level rises more slowly following intramuscular injection and a larger dose may be required to reach a therapeutic plasma concentration but, because of the continued uptake from muscle, the effective concentration may be maintained for longer. Variations in muscle blood flow (e.g. in shock where it is decreased) will result in similar variations in the rate of rise of plasma concentration. (b) A bolus injection will rapidly achieve a therapeutic plasma level which can then be maintained by an infusion (1). If a constant infusion is used from the start it will take some time to reach a therapeutic level. The high infusion concentration (3) will reach a therapeutic level more quickly and attain a higher steady state level than the lower infusion concentration (2).

The advent of long acting local anaesthetics (bupivacaine and etidocaine) have increased the use of regional blocks to provide postoperative analgesia. For example, intercostal blocks can be used for thoracic and upper abdominal surgery, a caudal can be used for circumcision or penile surgery and epidurals can be used for abdominal, perineal or thoracic surgery. The use of catheters placed in the epidural space allows repeated doses of local anaesthesia to be used so that the patient can be pain free for a day or two.

Special cases

(a) *Tracheostomy*

A tracheostomy can be performed to relieve upper airway obstruction, to ensure an adequate airway in patients who are difficult to intubate or who are having major head and neck surgery, to reduce dead space in patients with borderline respiratory insufficiency or who require prolonged ventilation and to provide tracheobronchial toilet in patients with prolonged unconsciousness following head injury.

In some of these circumstances a nasotracheal tube can be used to provide an artificial airway especially if only for a short time. Nasotracheal intubation has been more widely used in children than in adults because they are well tolerated and the correct size of tube for the larynx fits the nasal airway comfortably.

The problems with a recently performed tracheostomy include dislodgement of the tube, placement in a false tract, subcutaneous emphysema or pneumothorax (especially in small children) and blockage of the tube with secretions or blood (Fig. 8.3). A tracheostomy introducer should be available to replace a tube which is dislodged or has to be removed because it is in the wrong place or is blocked. Blockage of the tube is usually prevented by regular suction with a sterile catheter and humidification of the inspired air or oxygen.

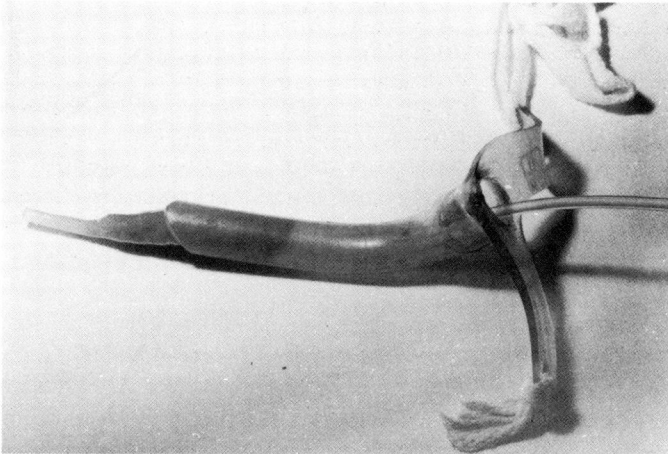

Fig. 8.3 A tracheotomy tube which was removed because it was blocked with thick secretions. Note that a fine suction catheter can pass through viscid secretions without necessarily removing them adequately. Adequate humidification and regular suctioning helps to prevent this problem.

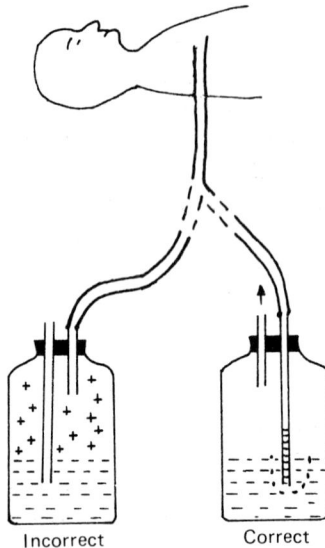

Incorrect   Correct

Fig. 8.4 Chest drain connection to the patient. The tube from the patient should be placed under water so that air in the chest can escape. The incorrect arrangement allows air to be sucked into the bottle where it creates a positive pressure which can be transmitted to the patient causing a tension pneumothorax.

(b) *Post-thoracotomy patients*

These patients usually have a chest drain (Fig. 8.4) which allows air to escape from the chest but not to enter the chest. This is achieved by placing the tube connected to the chest drain under water. Air in the chest can bubble off passively when intrathoracic pressure exceeds the amount the drain tube is placed under water (usually about 5 cm water) or gentle suction can be applied to the second tube in the bottle which is placed *above* water level.

The patient is usually placed with the operative side up because it is more comfortable, allows postural drainage of secretions from the operative side and is not splinted as much. Postoperative analgesia is important so that the patient can be encouraged to deep breathe and cough as soon as possible after surgery so that postoperative atelectasis is minimized. Intercostal nerve blocks of thoracic epidural block provides effective analgesia.

Oxygen should always be given to these patients as lung function is usually disturbed.

(c) *Recovery from ketamine*

This drug used mostly in burnt patients can cause unpleasant dreams, hallucinations and psychological disturbances. These undesirable effects are lessened if patients are allowed to recover without being disturbed. This contrasts with the usual approach to recovery where patients are roused to check on their conscious state and recovery. Laryngeal reflexes and muscle tone are retained with ketamine so that airway obstruction is unlikely during recovery.

Staff and responsibilities

The recovery room should be staffed with competent nurses who are skilled in airway management and in observing clinical signs. They have a great responsibility taking over the care of patients recovering consciousness following anaesthesia. Life threatening complications can develop rapidly and must be recognized and treated promptly if catastrophies are to be avoided. There should be enough staff to monitor all the patients frequently and cope with complications. The patients should be placed facing the direction from which they can be most easily watched by the staff. If the recovery room is fairly quiet and the patients are in a stable condition the nurses should still remain beside the patients rather than watch them from the central desk area. If desired stools can be moved adjacent to the patients (Fig. 8.5).

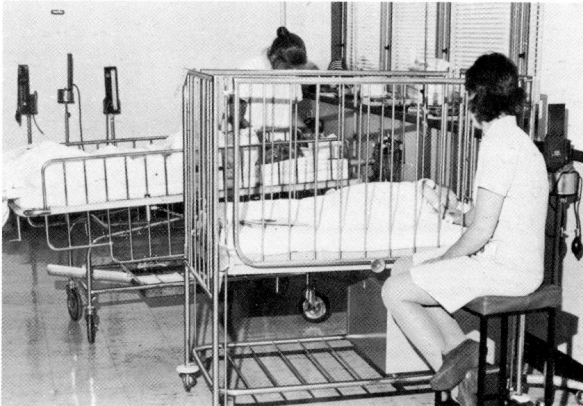

Fig. 8.5 Complications in the recovery room can occur at any time. They are more common if the patient is facing away from the staff. If stools are available for the nurses to sit on they should be placed beside the patients.

It is desirable to have an anaesthetist available nearby in case complications develop. A system for obtaining expert help rapidly should be organized so that staff do not have to leave the recovery room when they are most needed. Postoperative orders, including those for analgesia, should be completed and returned to the recovery room with the patient so that nurses do not have to waste time obtaining them and therefore not being available for patient care.

Returning to the ward

When the patient is fully conscious and in a stable condition he can be taken back to the ward. The orderly or porter should be accompanied by a nurse, preferably from the ward.

Complications occasionally occur even after the patient returns to the ward so that continuing observation of pulse, blood pressure, respiration and general appearance of the patient is necessary.

CHAPTER 9

Electrical hazards and safety in the operating theatre

By Mr Glen Johnston

Electromedical safety

Various items of electrical equipment are commonly used in operating theatres. These include surgical equipment such as diathermy and various endoscopes (bronchoscopes, cystoscopes etc); monitoring equipment such as ECG, pressure and temperature monitoring devices; patient support systems such as electrically driven ventilators, heart lung machines and electronic heart pacing devices; and a variety of other specialized diagnostic aids.

In the past before electrical equipment was widely used the main hazard was from fire and explosions of flammable anaesthetic agents such as ether and cyclopropane. Because static electricity was a potential cause of ignition special conductive floors were installed, anaesthetic machines had chains to earth them to the floor and antistatic rubber was used in anaesthetic circuits. The increasing use of electrical equipment and the introduction of better non-flammable anaesthetic agents has led to the virtual disappearance of cyclopropane and ether from anaesthetic practice in many places.

The main hazard associated with the use of electrical equipment now is electrocution with the potential for causing burns or ventricular

fibrillation. Patients who are anaesthetized, heavily sedated or unconscious may not respond normally to electric shock or heat so that these
complications may not be immediately recognized.

It is important that people working in operating theatres and adjacent
areas should be aware of the potential electrical hazards and the precautions that should be taken with electrical equipment so that maximum safety is provided for the patients and theatre personnel.

Basic physics of electricity

Some basic electrical knowledge is desirable before considering the
hazards of electric shock and electrocution and the precautions to be
observed when electromedical equipment is used.

The three fundamental elements of any electrical circuit are the
voltage, or electrical pressure applied, the resistance of the material
concerned and the current or flow which results. The relationship
between these three elements is expressed in Ohm's Law which says
that

$$\text{I (current)} = \frac{\text{V (voltage applied)}}{\text{R (resistance)}}$$

or conversely $$V = IR, \quad R = \frac{V}{I}$$

The basic unit of current is the ampere, but in electromedical
applications, it is frequently necessary to employ smaller units such as
the milliamp (amperes/1000) or even the microampere (amperes/
1 000 000).

The basic unit of electrical pressure is the volt. The AC mains supply
is usually 240 v and an ordinary torch battery provides a nominal 1.4
volts. In patient situations, much smaller voltages (millivolts or even
microvolts) may be significant.

The basic unit of resistance is the ohm. Good conductors including
metals, especially copper, have low resistances. Body tissue and blood are
good conductors, but the human skin, if dry, offers high resistance to
current flow.

Electric shock and electrocution

The most common hazard in hospitals is equipment operating from the
50 Hz (cycle/s) AC mains supply and the supply itself.

(a) *Physiological effects of varying current intensity*

The amount of current and the time of application determine the effect on the body. Table 9.1 summarizes approximately the effect produced by a 1s skin contact of various currents.

Table 9.1   Effects of increasing current intensity.

Current intensity maintained for 1s	Effect
1 mA	Threshold of perception
5 mA	Maximum harmless intensity
10–20 mA	Limit of 'let-go' current before sustained muscular contraction
50 mA	Pain, possible fainting, exhaustion, mechanical injury. Heart and respiratory functions continue
80–130 mA	Onset of ventricular fibrillation. Respiratory centre remains intact

(b) *Current density*

Current density relates the amount of current to the area to which it is applied. A given current produces a greater effect when applied to a small area than a larger area. The patient (or indifferent) electrode of the diathermy (see later) is large to minimize current density and heating while the active electrode is small so that heat is produced for cutting and coagulation.

Sources of electric shock

Some hazard exists every time a patient is attached to a piece of electrical equipment. There are several possible sources of current.

1   The apparatus may provide a source of current which may enter the patient via the patient connection, e.g. leakage current which occurs in all equipment even when operating normally. A *fault* current occurs when there is an abnormal insulation breakdown in the apparatus.

2   The apparatus and its patient circuit may provide a return path for a current originating from *another source* such as leakage or fault current from another piece of equipment attached to the patient.

3   Chassis (or enclosure) leakage. The patient may accidentally contact the exposed metal enclosure or chassis of a nearby piece of electrical equipment thus providing a path to earth for its leakage current.

Modes of shock

(a) *Macroshocks*
These are produced by currents of 80–300 m amps or more applied to the external surface of the body. Currents in this range may cause ventricular fibrillation while lower currents may shock or burn.

(b) *Microshock*
Microshock is a very low current (as low as 30 μ amps) at low voltage (3–5 mv) which can cause fibrillation if applied directly to the heart or through electrical connections within the thorax and extending out through the body surface (e.g. via pacing leads, transvenous pacing catheters, saline filled pressure cannulae etc.) — (Fig. 9.1).

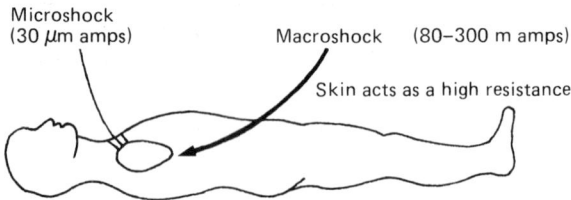

Microshock
(30 μm amps)   Macroshock   (80–300 m amps)
                    Skin acts as a high resistance

Fig. 9.1   This illustrates the very small current required to cause ventricular fibrillation when there is direct access to the heart (microshock) compared to the much greater current required when applied to the surface to overcome skin and tissue resistance (macroshock).

Equipment classification

Electrical equipment used for patient care is classified according to the level of patient protection provided. Class A equipment limits the current which may pass between the equipment and the patient to 10 μ amps. It is suitable for use with patients having electrical connection within the thorax, and therefore susceptible to microshock. Class B equipment provides less protection. It limits the passage of current in the patient circuit to 100 μ amps. Class Z is similar to class B but allows an earth connection to the patient's body. It is not now recommended for connection to patients.

Earth connection

It was formerly thought to be good practice to make an efficient earth connection to a patient's body. This is no longer the case.

The mains supply is carried by two wires — the so-called 'active' or live wire, and the 'neutral' which is connected to earth. Any earth made to the patient's body therefore represents a connection to one side of the mains supply and an inadvertent, or leakage path to the other side of the supply may complete a hazardous or even fatal circuit. The danger is considerably increased by the attachment of multiple earth connections to the patient because of the multiplicity of possible leakage paths created. The main risk is that the normal equipment leakage current can return to earth via the patient's body and a second earth circuit.

The other problem is that there may be a potential difference between any two earth points, due to different resistances back to the earth reference or the two earth circuits carrying different leakage currents. The hazards related to different earth potentials are overcome by (a) the installation of a heavy gauge copper cable between the earth points of all power outlets to produce an equipotential earth (or equipotential patient reference, EPR) system and (b) wiring the patient care areas so that only the loads from within a given area are carried by the earthing and earth equalizing system for that area.

Environmental protection

All areas in hospitals where electromedical equipment is regularly used for patient procedures classified as class A or class B must provide protection against macroshock. The two methods used are (a) core balance relay which prevents excessive leakage current and cuts off power in the event of earth leakage and (b) an isolation transformer which only activates an audible-visual warning if excessive leakage occurs.

All areas where class A procedures are performed must provide protection against microshock. This is achieved by the installation of an equipotential patient reference (EPR) system (see Earth Connection above).

Marking of classified areas and equipment

(a) *Environment*
Those areas of a hospital in which elevated levels of environmental electrical protection have been installed are suitably marked by a prominent notice, usually positioned slightly above eye level to indicate the status of the area, e.g. 'Class A electrical area' or 'Class B electrical area'. The lettering of the sign will be white on a green background.

Those areas not so marked should be presumed to afford no special level of patient protection.

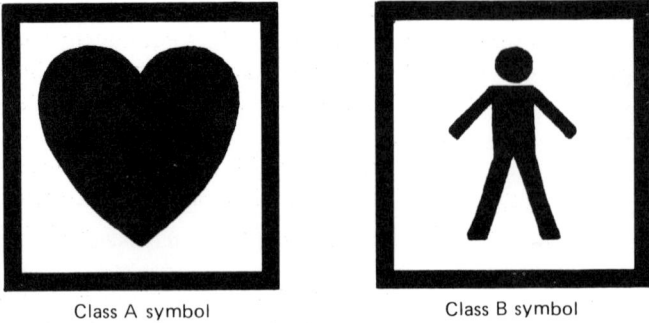

Class A symbol   Class B symbol

Fig. 9.2 Labels used on patient care equipment to indicate the patient safety classification.

(b) *Equipment*
Equipment providing patient protection of class A or B levels should have the appropriate symbol (Fig. 9.2) attached adjacent to the patient circuit connector which is usually on the front of the apparatus.

On class A equipment the same symbol may also appear near the manufacturer's rating plate on the back of the equipment. This refers to the enclosure chassis leakage current and signifies an adequate level of protection (class A) should the patient accidentally touch the equipment or be connected to it by someone touching the patient and the equipment at the same time.

General precautions

1   Before using any piece of patient-care equipment, ascertain whether it is the right class for the procedure concerned.
2   Remember that an intact earth-wire in the mains power lead is the patient's greatest protection. Before connecting any piece of equipment to a patient, *always* examine the power lead carefully for (a) positive connection of all three wires at the power plug and (b) evidence of damage to the outer insulating sheath which might suggest interruption of any of the three inner wires. Do not connect any equipment which fails this examination.
3   Never leave a malfunctioning monitor connected to a patient. It may provide an earth or other leakage path. If the usual checks fail to restore it to working order, switch it off, and remove the power plug from the wall outlet. Remove the patient connections (e.g. electrodes, temperature probe, pressure cannula) as soon as practicable.

4 The presence of an unexplained and persistent interference pattern on an ECG monitor may be an indication of an equipment fault or a poorly attached electrode. On the other hand it may well indicate an excessive level of 50 Hz (50 cycle/s) AC signal in the patient's body, requiring immediate investigation.

5 It is undesirable that non-technical staff should attempt the replacement of fuses in patient-care instrumentation. Should this be necessary in an emergency, first switch the unit *off* and remove the plug from the wall outlet.

6 Do not place intravenous bottles or other fluids on top of monitoring or other electrical equipment. Sooner or later, spillage will occur, and protective insulation may be bypassed. Never mop up spilt liquid from on or within a mains-operated instrument without first disconnecting the mains lead from the wall outlet.

7 Never cover equipment ventilation holes or grilles with drapes, towels, bowls or other equipment. They are essential to the instrument's cooling arrangements. Overheating may result in component failure, the breakdown of protective insulation, or even a fire.

8 Except in emergency circumstances, do not use power extension leads. The incorrect wiring of such a lead may have fatal consequences. If the mains lead on any piece of apparatus is not long enough for its normal location it should be replaced with a single lead of appropriate length.

9 In certain areas of hospitals, notably operating theatres, the floors are deliberately earthed. In all areas, the floors must be presumed to be at earth potential. Remember that your body is an electrical conductor, and that every time you place a hand on a patient, you effectively apply an earth connection to that point of contact. This is especially so if the other hand is in contact with a deliberately-earthed piece of equipment.

10 Be aware constantly of the two-fold aim of all patient electrical safety procedures: the isolation (or insulation) of the patient from the active supply, and from earth. *Both are hazardous.*

Diathermy

Diathermy is the use of radiofrequency current for cutting tissues and coagulation of blood vessels. It is a commonly employed and useful technique in surgery but its use is associated with more accidents than with any other class of electromedical equipment. It is important that all members of theatre staff understand its hazards and are familiar with the precautions necessary for its safe use.

Cutting

The fundamental principle in the cutting mode is that an electric arc is struck between the point of the 'active' electrode attached to the surgeon's handpiece and the patient's tissue. The temperature of the arc may exceed 1000°C and is sufficient to part the tissues like a knife. The power required for cutting tissues is about three times that required for coagulation using traditional monopolar methods. (Power is measured in watts. Watts = volts × amps.)

Monopolar diathermy has a small area 'active' electrode applied at the site of surgery producing a high current density, high temperature and, therefore, the ability to cut and coagulate. It also has a large area 'indifferent' electrode (often referred to colloquially as the 'diathermy plate') in close contact with the patient's skin (Fig. 9.3). Because the total current remains the same throughout the circuit the current density at the indifferent electrode is low, provided there is good skin contact, because of the large surface area. To ensure good contact a conductive paste or gel is used (or a saline soaked pack). Care must be taken *not* to use KY jelly and other lubricants which have insulating rather than conducting properties. If the indifferent patient electrode does not make good contact with the skin and the contact area is reduced the current density increases and tissue damage and burns may result. If the 'indifferent' patient electrode is not connected to the machine or its cable is broken the current must be dissipated by another route, for example via an ECG earth lead (Fig. 9.4). This may have a small surface area so that a high current density develops with the likelihood of burning the skin. It

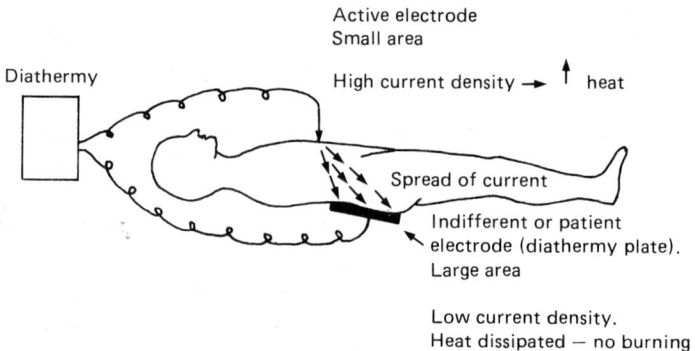

Fig. 9.3 Monopolar diathermy. The spread of current in the body from a discrete active monopolar electrode to the larger indifferent electrode (diathermy plate).

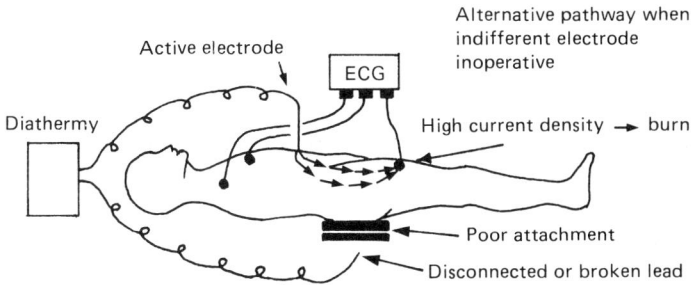

Fig. 9.4 If the indifferent electrode connection to the patient is unsatisfactory, there is a potential hazard of burns.

is of the utmost importance to ensure the continuity of the indifferent circuit and its attachment to the patient is satisfactory.

The first indication of an unsatisfactory indifferent connection is inefficient diathermy performance, a condition which may prompt the surgeon to request an increase in power output. *Under no circumstances* should such a request be granted until the indifferent circuit has been checked and found to be intact.

Coagulation

Coagulation, using monopolar diathermy, is achieved by clamping the open end of the blood vessel with an artery forceps and applying the diathermy current to it for a brief period.

The problem with monopolar coagulation is that the operator cannot control how the current spreads from the contact point apart from adjusting the power source. For delicate and precise surgical procedures (e.g. in surgery on the brain or spinal cord) the more recently introduced bipolar technique has overcome this problem. It employs the application of a small current between two small electrodes of equal area which are often the tips of a pair of insulated surgical forceps (Fig. 9.5). Neither electrode is active or indifferent and the effect achieved is identical in both. The small mass of tissue through which the current passes and the low power output required from the generator, which can be accurately controlled, allow precision in coagulation not possible with the monopolar technique. Cutting is not possible with the bipolar mode.

The diathermy is usually activated by foot or hand switches which allow cutting, coagulating or a blending of the two. Some makes of

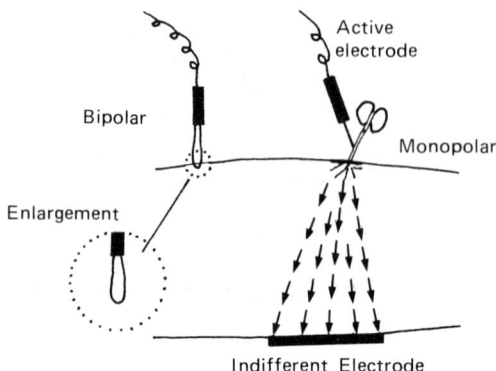

Fig. 9.5 Coagulation. The discrete coagulation with the bipolar compared with the monopolar mode.

generator provide only monopolar or bipolar output but most modern generators provide both. Since activating one, by a hand or foot switch, usually means generation of current in both, special care must be observed by the surgical team when both types of output are connected. All 'active' monopolar and bipolar electrodes should be kept in an insulating holster when not in use to avoid accidental burning.

Earthing

Formerly the patient or indifferent side of the diathermy output circuit was earthed at the generator. Recently it has been realized that any earth connection on the patient's body is hazardous and undesirable. Earthing of the patient side of the output circuit is hazardous because any interruption of it allows any other earth connection on the patient's body to provide a return path for the diathermy current. Should this other earth connection have a small area of contact, high current density may develop with the risk of burning. In no circumstances, where solidly earthed or 'non-isolated' diathermy is in use, should a further earth connection be made to the patient. For example, this may be the earthed electrode (RL) of an earth-referenced ECG monitor. This electrode should be connected to the diathermy indifferent electrode ('patient diathermy plate') rather than to the patient (Fig. 9.6).

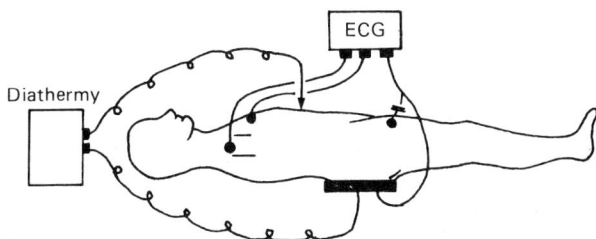

Fig. 9.6 ECG earth lead attached to patient indifferent electrode.

General precautions with the use of diathermy

The following points are significant in the safe and efficient use of surgical diathermy.

1 As with any other piece of electromedical equipment, the most important single item in ensuring the safety of both patient and theatre staff is the continuity of the earth (green and yellow) wire in the three-wire mains cable of the generator. Whoever is delegated to plug the unit in, *must* examine the three-pin plug to see that all three wires are securely terminated, a condition readily checked through a clear-backed plug.

2 Examine the outer insulating sheath of the power cable along the whole of its length for damage. If there is any evidence to suggest that any one of the inner conductors, or its insulation, has been damaged the generator should be put aside for checking by competent maintenance personnel.

3 Examine the indifferent lead throughout its length and at its termination at the indifferent electrode. Theatre staff frequently fold the lead around the plate between use. Consistent folding of the lead in the same place and occasional autoclaving, will eventually corrode, fatigue and fracture the individual conductors of the wire in the lead. Regular use of a simple continuity testing device is recommended.

4 Use an indifferent electrode which makes a large area contact with the body surface and see that it is positioned on an area with a generous thickness of tissue. High current density and burning, or simply pressure damage, may develop over an area where bone is covered with a minimum thickness of tissue. Subcutaneous adipose fat is not a good conductor of heat and may prevent the dispersion of surface heat into lower layers of tissue.

5 Always use a good-quality, non-migrating gel to provide a low-resistance interface between electrode and tissue. KY jelly and other lubricants have insulating rather than conducting qualities and should *not* be used. Packs saturated in saline, sometimes 20 times isotonic, are frequently wrapped around malleable plates to provide a conducting interface. Their conducting qualities deteriorate as the water evaporates in a warm theatre during a long procedure.

6 When using an earth referenced diathermy make sure that the indifferent electrode is the only earth connection on the patient's body. Connect all other earths to the plate and not to the patient.

7 Place the indifferent electrode as close as practicable to the surgical site.

8 Use the minimum generator output power which will satisfactorily perform the functions required. Treat a request for increased power output, above the level commonly used for a given application, as an indication of a possible fault condition in either the generator or the patient circuit.

9 Dress the leads on both sides of the output circuit well clear of body tissue. Where either lead lies in close proximity to tissue, sufficient capacity may exist to transfer enough radio-frequency energy to cause a burn in a small contact area. The active lead to the surgeon's handpiece should be under direct surveillance throughout its length, but the indifferent lead, particularly in the vicinity of the indifferent electrode, is frequently hidden by surgical drapes. It should be dressed to run at least 5 cm clear of the patient's body throughout the whole length of its run and taped in position to prevent inadvertent movement after the drapes have been placed.

10 An insulated holster should be provided for every diathermy procedure to hold all active electrodes when not actually in use.

11 The positioning and attachment of the indifferent electrode are of vital importance to the efficient performance of the diathermy system, as well as to the safety of the patient.

Despite an inevitable impatience to get the operation started, a few moments of cool deliberation about the location of the indifferent electrode, its secure attachment and the dress and connection of its lead are essential in the interests of both patient and staff.

Laser radiation

Lasers are becoming more widely used in surgery and a knowledge of their hazards is desirable. Many lasers are capable of inflicting biological damage. For most laser wavelengths this damage occurs principally through the heat generated by the interaction of light with matter. Ultraviolet light generated by lasers will interact directly with organic molecules to cause cell damage in addition to the heat mechanism of damage. Very high power lasers may also produce a thermally induced shock wave which may harm tissue some distance from the site of beam exposure by physical displacement of the tissue.

In addition to the hazards of exposure to the direct laser beam, exposure to its specular reflections caused by smooth reflecting surfaces such as mirrors, lenses, untreated surgical instruments and so on is often hazardous depending upon the amount of electromagnetic energy reflected. Diffuse reflections may also be hazardous when the reflected electromagnetic energy is sufficiently intense. The eye and the skin are the most susceptible parts of the body for laser injury. Glasses should be worn by everyone in the theatre to protect their eyes.

The other hazard of lasers, especially when used in the airways, is the potential for setting plastic tubes on fire. This can be reduced by covering the tube with foil, by protecting from direct exposure using wet swabs or patties and by avoiding 100% oxygen in the inspired gas. The surgeon will make every effort to avoid striking the tube directly or indirectly with the laser.

APPENDIX 1

Cardiac and respiratory arrest

Consequences of cardiac arrest. Causes. Recognition. Action to be taken. Assessment of progress. Summary of management and roles to be fulfilled. The basic management of a person who collapses.

Cardiac arrest is the cessation of an effective heart beat. Anaesthetists, particularly those involved in intensive care, are frequently called when a cardiac arrest occurs in hospital because of their expertise with ventilation and resuscitation. They often provide instruction to the staff on the management of cardiac arrest. Medical students often gain practical experience during their anaesthetic term of intubation and ventilation which is essential in cardiopulmonary resuscitation. This appendix outlines the procedures for cardiopulmonary resuscitation in hospital although the basic principles apply anywhere.

Consequences of cardiac arrest

The consequences of cardiac arrest are that the heart stops pumping blood around the body, the oxygen supply to the tissues ceases and the available oxygen is rapidly used up for metabolism. The brain is dependent on oxygen which it utilizes rapidly. Available oxygen in the brain is used up in about 3 minutes after circulator arrest. Hypoxic brain damage or death will occur if the oxygen supply is not promptly re-established. If the arrest is not recognized immediately some or all of the oxygen reserve may have been used up before resuscitation begins. No time can therefore be wasted.

The lack of oxygen in the tissues leads to anaerobic metabolism with the production of carbon dioxide and acid metabolites. This causes a metabolic and respiratory acidosis and a fall in pH (see Acid Base Balance, Chapter 4).

Causes

Cardiac arrest may result from primary heart disease or the heart may fail as a consequence of tissue hypoxia resulting from respiratory failure, blood loss, shock or overdosage with drugs which depress the heart and adversely affect cardiac output. The causes of respiratory failure are summarized on an anatomical basis in Fig. A1.1.

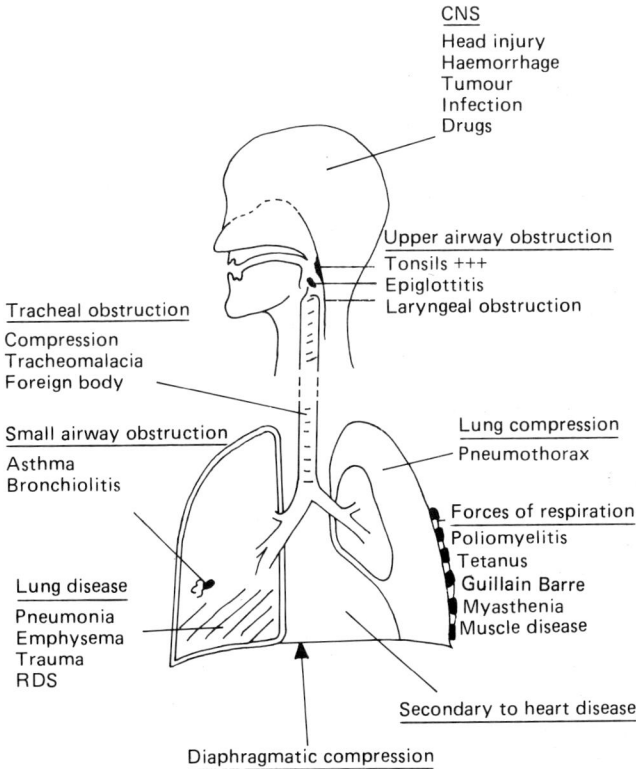

Fig. A1.1 Aetiology of respiratory failure. A diagrammatic representation of the anatomical classification of the commoner causes of respiratory failure.

Recognition

The patient collapses or, if in bed, becomes flaccid, stops breathing and becomes cyanosed (turns blue or pallid grey due to the lack of flow of oxygenated blood).

The pulse cannot be felt at any of the usual sites — the radial artery at the wrist, the brachial artery at the elbow, the axillary artery in the axilla, the carotid artery in the neck or the femoral artery in the groin. If the pulse cannot be felt easily at the wrist a larger artery is palpated or the hand can be put on the chest to feel for the heart beat. Do not spend time trying to feel a pulse which may not be there. Absence of a pulse can be confirmed by listening to the heart with a stethoscope (or with an ear on the chest if a stethoscope is not available).

Action to be taken

As soon as a cardiac arrest is suspected or recognized call for help and get someone to telephone for the hospital resuscitation team. It is desirable to segregate the patient from other patients in the ward by either pulling curtains around the bed or sometimes, especially in the case of a child, it is possible to transfer the patient rapidly to the ward treatment room.

The resuscitation routine should be begun as soon as possible and continued with as little interruption as possible until the patient recovers or treatment is discontinued.

1   The airway should be cleared by suction or manual removal of debris if present but it may only require extending the head and pulling the jaw forward thereby lifting the tongue off the posterior wall of the pharynx. An oral airway can be inserted if available.

2   Ventilation can then be achieved either by: (a) mouth to mouth expired air breathing (Fig. A1.2); (b) the use of a double airway (Fig. A1.3); (c) inflation with a self inflating bag (e.g. Ambu, Laerdal or Air viva, Fig. A1.4); (d) administration of oxygen with a mask or via an endotracheal tube. Time should not be spent attempting intubation until the patient has been ventilated adequately by mask. Time spent by unskilled people attempting to intubate unsuccessfully can aggravate hypoxia and lead to death. Added oxygen using (c) and (d) should be used whenever possible.

3   Cardiac massage is achieved by intermittent compression with two hands crossed on the lower sternum (Fig. A1.5). It is usually compressed at a rate comparable to the normal heart rate (72/minute). A board is

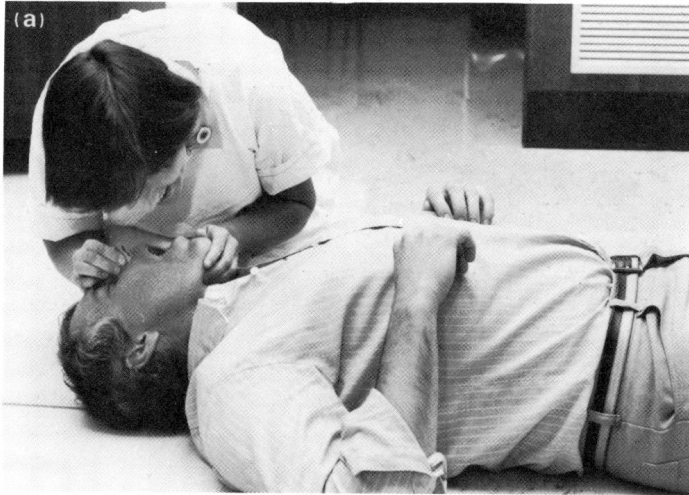

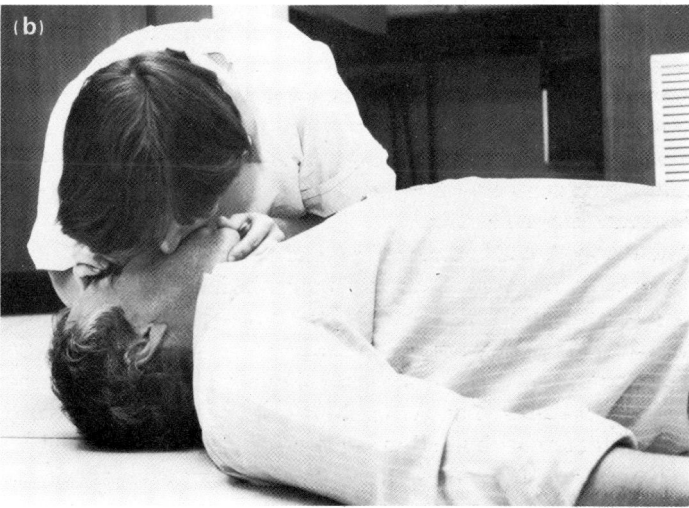

Fig. A1.2 Mouth to mouth resuscitation. The patient's mouth is opened and the airway cleared (a) before the resuscitator blows expired air into the patient (b) *Note.* These pictures demonstrate a common error in technique. The fingers have been placed under the chin where compression pushes the tongue upwards thus obstructing the airway. The fingers should be placed on the mandible so that they pull it forward. The nose is pinched with the other hand.

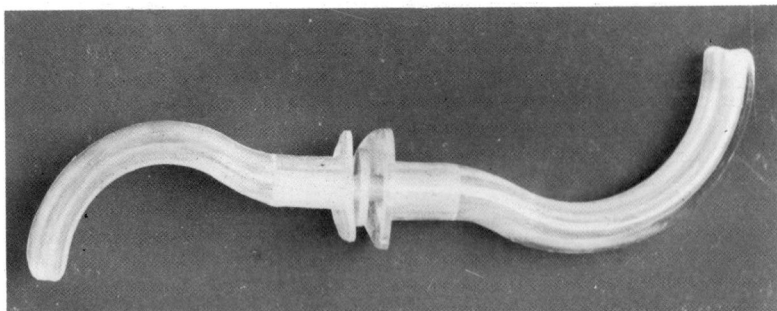

Fig. A1.3 Double airway. One end is placed in the patient's mouth and provides an airway while the resuscitator can blow into the other end.

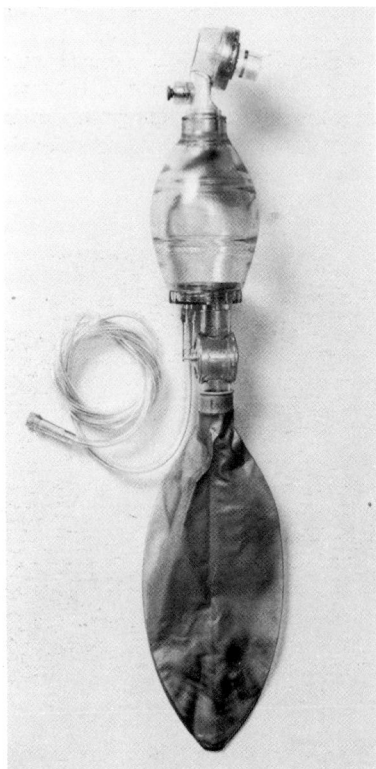

Fig. A1.4 The Laerdal bag is one variety of the self-inflating bag used in resuscitation.

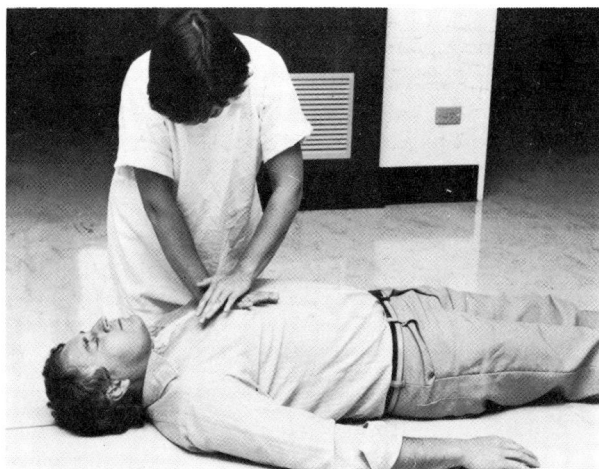

Fig. A1.5   Cardiac massage. The heel of one hand should be placed over the middle of the lower half of the sternum. The other hand is placed on top and the sternum is compressed (about 40 mm) keeping the arms straight. The patient should be on a firm surface (a board can be placed under him if in bed or he can be placed on the ground as shown here).

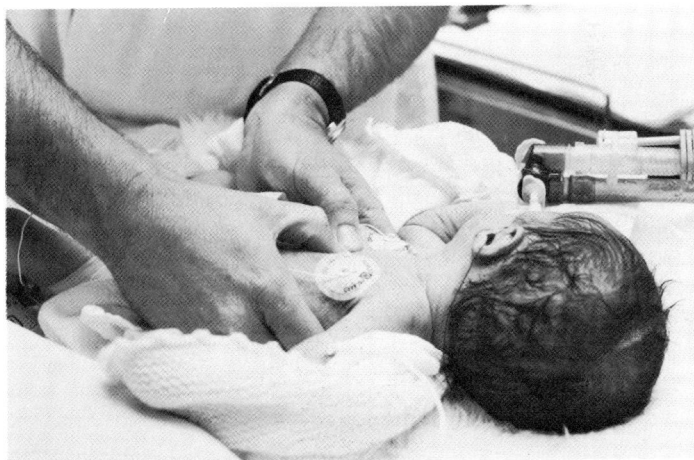

Fig. A1.6   Cardiac massage in infants. The heart can be compressed by the thumbs on the mid sternum while the back is supported by the fingers. Alternatively, if the baby is lying on a firm surface, the sternum can be compressed (about 12 mm) by two fingers.

usually placed under the patient to provide a firm base against which to depress the sternum to achieve cardiac output. Even the most efficient cardiac massage may only produce 30–50% of normal cardiac output.

In infants cardiac massage can be achieved with one or more fingers of one hand compressing the sternum about 25 mm or alternatively the thumb can compress the sternum with the fingers supporting the back (Fig. A1.6). (Rate 100–120/minute.)

If one is alone at an arrest the one man arrest pattern of resuscitation should be instituted. In adults two breaths are given followed by 15 cardiac compressions and the cycle is then repeated. In children four breaths are followed by 20 more rapid cardiac compressions.

When two people are available one should ventilate the patient and the other undertake the cardiac massage giving one breath for every fifth compression of the heart. It is now recommended that cardiac massage should be a continuous regular pattern even though this makes ventilation more difficult. Formerly massage was interrupted while the patient was inflated.

As soon as further assistance arrives the role of the nurse or assistant is to collect the resuscitative equipment (laryngoscope, endotracheal tubes, etc), drugs (adrenaline, sodium bicarbonate, calcium), syringes, needles and to set up an intravenous infusion set. If cardiac arrest occurs in the operating theatre the anaesthetic technician or nurse assistant should immediately bring these items and prepare them for immediate use.

Sodium bicarbonate is given to correct the metabolic acidosis. The initial dose is usually 1 mmol/kg (8.4% solution has 1 mmol/ml while a 5% solution has about 0.6 mmol/ml). Adrenaline will increase the rate and force of contraction of the heart and may initiate the heart beat when it stops in asystole. It is usually given in a 1:10 000 solution (1:1000 should be diluted in 10 ml of saline) in a dose of up to 10 ml initially. Children are usually given about 1 ml/year.

When available an ECG is recorded. If ventricular fibrillation is present DC countershock is applied from a defibrillator usually after sodium bicarbonate has been given (usually 300–400 joules for an adult and 5 joules/kg in a child). When DC countershock is used an anti-arrhythmic drug is often given to stabilize the rhythm after the shock. Lignocaine is most commonly used (1 mg/kg followed by an infusion run at 2–4 mg/min in an adult).

Calcium chloride up to 5 mmol may be given *slowly* intravenously when myocardial contractility remains ineffective despite correction of hypoxia and acidosis.

In children cardiac arrest is usually in asystole unless there is myocardial disease. The administration of sodium bicarbonate and adrenaline together with adequate ventilation and massage will usually restart the heart. If it does not restart quickly the outcome is not likely to be successful. The successful treatment of patients with hypovolaema or shock requires concurrent blood volume replacement to maintain an effective cardiac output.

Overdosage with depressant drugs will require ventilation for respiratory arrest and a myocardial stimulant such as adrenaline or isoprenaline to overcome the drug induced myocardial depression.

Assessment of progress

The effectiveness of resuscitation must be continually reassessed. Improvement in colour, the return of a palpable pulse and measurable blood pressure, a normal ECG pattern and the return of spontaneous respiration are all promising signs. Auscultation of the heart sounds is useful, especially in children, as the intensity of the sounds gives some indication of cardiac output, being soft when it is poor and loud when it is satisfactory.

Summary of management

The routine management of cardiac arrest can be summarized as follows:
1 Airway — clear it.
2 Breathing — start it (stop bleeding if obvious).
3 Circulation — restore it.
  The roles to be undertaken are as follows:
1 Call for help.
2 Clear the airway and ventilate the patient.
3 Cardiac massage.
4 Prepare resuscitation equipment and drugs for use.
5 Set up an intravenous infusion.
6 Record the drugs given and doses.
7 Record fluids given and volumes.
8 Record the ECG and, if necessary, defibrillate the patient.
  Work down the list as help arrives so that eventually all steps will be undertaken. When the resuscitation team arrives they will usually take

over ventilation, cardiac massage, the insertion of an intravenous drip, the administration of drugs and defibrillation if required. The nurses or assistants can then play an important role organizing suction if required, assisting with intubation, supplying the drugs and fluids to whoever is giving them and recording what is given. If cardiac resuscitation is to be successful it must be applied promptly and carried on continuously until recovery. The multiple roles that have to be fulfilled require several people if they are to be undertaken efficiently and effectively. Those helping fulfil a vital role.

The basic management of the person who collapses

There are many causes of collapse. The important steps on coming across a collapsed person are to (a) turn the patient on the side, check the airway and clear it if necessary, (b) if the patient is breathing leave on side and keep airway clear, if not begin mouth to mouth ventilation, (c) if the pulse is absent begin cardiac massage and (d) call for help or get someone to call for an ambulance.

APPENDIX 2

Procedures in relation to anaesthesia for handling infected patients

Objectives. Patients and operations defined as septic or infected. Preoperative and preanaesthetic procedures. During the anaesthetic. At the completion of the anaesthetic.

Special procedures have been developed in operating theatres to minimize contamination by infected material (e.g. pus) or patients and for cleaning the theatres after 'dirty' cases so that following patients do not become infected. Although the cleaning procedures are basically the same some septic (or 'dirty') cases present a greater hazard of contamination — spread of infection due to the organism involved being more virulent (e.g. *Staphyloccus aureus*) or more resistant to decontamination (e.g. tuberculosis). Basic procedures are outlined in this section for handling anaesthetic equipment.

Objectives

1   To protect other patients and the staff handling the patient.
2   To prevent the spread of bacteria to other areas from the focal area.
3   To provide a safe, clean and pathogen free operating theatre for the next patient.

Patients and operations defined as septic or infected

1   The presence of pus in a cavity or wound.
2   Operations involving the opening of bowel.
3   All rectal surgery.
4   Infected with gas gangrene.

5 Tuberculous patients.
6 Patients with chronic infections such as MRSA (multiple resistant *Staphyloccus aureus*) and hepatitis.

Definitions 2 and 3 are surgically potentially contaminated but create less hazard to the anaesthetic equipment.

Preoperative and preanaesthetic procedure

The basic aim is to plan what equipment will be required for the infected patient and remove all other equipment.
1 Remove all mobile equipment from the anaesthetic room and place in a storage or holding area, e.g. scrub room (placing equipment so that access to the holding room can be maintained).
2 Cover with double drape any equipment that cannot be removed.
3 Strip the anaesthetic machine of all equipment not needed for that particular case.
4 Place a plastic disposable bag in readiness to receive contaminated rubbish. When placing this bag ensure that it is opened out so that contaminated items do not contact the outside of the bag.
5 Prepare an area on the sink bench for contaminated items other than rubbish.
6 Place trays or basket on the bench to receive the articles suitable for steam sterilization.
7 Have a soaking dish for chemical disinfection of items unable to be steam sterilized.
8 Have a brown paper bag marked 'contaminated anaesthetic items' for gamma sterilization.
9 Prepare a clean gown, disposable gloves, cleaning cloths and cleaning solution of chemical suitable for disinfection in readiness for the clean up.
10 Have a bowl of disinfectant and a scrub brush on hand to wash surface dirt off items for sterilization or disinfection.

During the anaesthetic

1 A gown and gloves should be worn when handling infected patients.
2 Any item used during the anaesthetic should be placed in a receiver prepared for its disposal.

3   Linen is discarded into the contaminated linen bag prepared in theatre.

At the completion of the anaesthetic

1   When the anaesthetic is over and the patient's condition is satisfactory he is transferred to a trolley, covered with a warm towel and taken to the recovery room unless it has been decided that he would be a contamination hazard there. In that case the patient should be recovered in theatre until it is safe for him to return directly to his ward.

2   During this time the equipment used on this patient is placed into appropriate disposal areas within the theatre.

3   The gown and gloves are removed prior to transfer of the patient from the operating theatre.

4   The hands are thoroughly washed on return to the theatre area and a clean gown and gloves are donned.

5   The clean-up procedure is carried out by systematically going through and washing the used items for sterilization or disinfection, then placing them into their respective containers for sterilization.

6   Disinfectant is sucked through the suction tubing and nozzle into the sucker bottle.

7   The contaminated solution is discarded in a safe manner into a slop-hopper used for this purpose.

8   All items are then sterilized or disinfected. This includes the anaesthetic circuit which should be disassembled and disinfected or sterilized appropriately. In patients with pulmonary tuberculosis or infected with an organism which is very virulent or difficult to eradicate a disposable circuit can be used. A Water's to and from rebreathing circuit can be employed instead of a circle absorber system because it can be easily sterilized.

9   All exposed surfaces, including the anaesthetic machine, are cleaned with chemical disinfectant. Particular attention should be paid to cleaning the knobs for turning the rotameters and vapourizers on and off because the anaesthetist's gloved hands can become contaminated.

10   The floor should be washed.

When the clean-up is completed the unused equipment is returned to the anaesthetic room.

APPENDIX 3

The applications of Ohms law to physiology and flow of fluids

Ohms Law related current flow (I), resistance (R) and potential difference (V) in electricity (see Basic Physics of Electricity, Chapter 9) in the relationship $V = IR$. These can be substituted for fluids and gas flow:

Pressure = flow × resistance.

In cardiovascular physiology this becomes

Blood pressure = cardiac output × peripheral resistance.

In respiratory physiology resistance refers to airways resistance.

Resistance in relation to flow of fluids depends on and is proportional to the length of the tube and the viscosity of the fluid and inversely proportional to radius[4] (laminar flow) or radius[5] (turbulent flow) of the tubes (Poiseuille's equation).

These factors are important in the flow of fluids from intravenous sets or syringes and needles. A higher pressure is required to inject a given volume through a fine needle than a larger needle in a given time or it will take longer to inject through a fine bore needle if the pressure is constant.

Intravenous cannulae (and needles) vary in length. The longer the cannula the greater the resistance to flow. Flow through a cannula is faster than through a catheter of the same internal diameter.

If a fluid is viscous it will flow more slowly. For example, blood or 10% dextrose will flow more slowly than saline (0.9%) or 5% dextrose.

Hence, if a rapid intravenous infusion is required a short, large bore cannula should be used.

APPENDIX 4

Has this book achieved its aims?

Anaesthesia is a practical specialty which involves much applied pharmacology and physiology. It is hoped that having read this book you will have learnt the principles involved in caring for the safety and comfort of patients undergoing anaesthesia. The aims of the book were drawn up prior to writing it and are presented here as a series of broad questions which you can ask yourself to see whether you acquired the information which the book is aimed to present. Do you:

1 Appreciate how patients react to having an operation and the particular problems in children such as parental separation?

2 Understand the purpose of premedication and know why the various drugs are used?

3 Know what basic preoperative information is required by the anaesthetist and why this is necessary?

4 Know how to check the patient leaving the ward and arriving in theatre?

5 Know how to check the gas supplies and anaesthetic in the vaporizers on the machine?

6 Know the essential equipment that is set out for an anesthetic including the different sizes for children, e.g. laryngoscopes, tubes, masks, circuits?

7 Know the reasons for monitoring various physiological parameters, what monitoring aids are available and for what purpose they are used?

8 Know how and why the following basic groups of drugs are used in anaesthesia and understand their potential hazards? Induction agents, inhalation agents, muscle relaxants, analgesics and antagonists, atropine and neostigmine, local anaesthetics?

9 Know how to assist an anaesthetist at induction and the conclusion of anaesthesia?

10 Know how to set up an intravenous infusion and appreciate the factors which influence the choice of fluid and rate of infusion for intravenous fluids and blood?

11   Understand the principles of blood grouping and cross matching and the importance of correct identification and checking of blood before transfusion?

12   Appreciate the sources and causes of electrical hazards in the operating theatre and how these can be avoided?

13   Understand the principles of diathermy and the precautions to be taken when it is used?

14   In the recovery room, know how to determine that the patient is breathing adequately, what vital signs are checked and why, when to call for help and understand the reason why patients are usually positioned in the lateral position?

15   Know the basic steps to be taken if cardiac or respiratory arrest occur and know what drugs may be used and why?

BIBLIOGRAPHY

There are many texts available on anaesthesia and related topics. A few of these are mentioned here for those who want to read more widely.

Major textbooks

Evans F.T. and Gray T.C. *General Anaesthesia*. Butterworths, London.

Wylie W.D. and Churchill-Davidson H.C. *A Practice of Anaesthesia*. Lloyd-Luke.

Miller R.D. *Anesthesia*. Churchill Livingstone, Edinburgh.

Brown T.C.K. and Fisk G.C. *Anaesthesia for Children*. Blackwell Scientific Publications, Oxford.

Introductory books

Norris W. and Campbell D. *A Nurse's Guide to Anaesthetics, Resuscitation and Intensive Care*. Churchill Livingstone, Edinburgh.

Lunn J.N. *Lecture Notes on Anaesthetics*. Blackwell Scientific Publications, Oxford.

Dripps R.D., Eckenhoff J.E. and Vandam L.D. *Introduction to Anaesthesia*. W.B. Saunders, Philadelphia.

Foster C.A. and Jepson B. *Anaesthesia for Operating Theatre Technicians*. Lloyd Luke, London.

Equipment

Ward C.S. *Anaesthetic Equipment: physical principles and maintenance*. Bailliere Tindall, London.

Dorsch J.A. and Dorsch S.E. *Understanding Anesthesia Equipment: construction, care and complications*. Williams and Wilkins, Baltimore.

INDEX

151

5034